Nutritional
Harmony

The information presented is for educational purposes only and is not meant to replace consultations with a health care professional. The author/ publisher is not providing any form of counseling, professional advice or services (including diagnosis or treatment) to the reader. The information on nutrition including food, beverages, vitamins, nutrients, and supplements contained in this book does not cover all possible uses or mechanisms of action, does not cover precautions, does not cover possible interactions or side effects. The author/publisher is not liable or responsible for any individual actions, omissions, consequences, or medical outcomes that may occur based on the application of the information presented in this book. Never disregard professional health care advice or delay in seeking it because of the information presented in this book. Seek the advice of a physician or other qualified health care provider for all health care recommendations and concerns.

Nutritional Harmony

Tuning Your Diet to Cancer
And Chronic Disease Prevention

Christine Fall, MD, ABIHM

About *Nutritional Harmony*

In an age of rising disease and cancer, prevention can only be achieved by restoring harmony. The processing of food has destroyed the natural harmony that exists among the components of whole foods, removing the very nutrients necessary for disease prevention. Through *Nutritional Harmony* we begin to understand how the health of the gut and our pro-inflammatory diet promote heart disease, mood disorders, neurodegenerative diseases and cancer. We then learn how to use "food as medicine" with simple techniques for food selection and preparation. With an evidence based, scientific approach we see how these techniques have proven life saving benefits. *Nutritional Harmony* empowers us with the knowledge we need to reestablish harmony, restore our health, and ultimately prevent chronic disease and cancer.

To my family, whose love and support has allowed me to pursue my passions.

To my patients, who continue to inspire me in my pursuit of disease prevention and wellness.

Table of Contents

Chapter 1

Understanding Nutritional Harmony

Harmony comes from the Greek word, harmonia meaning "joint, agreement, concord".[1] In music, harmony refers to the combination of two or more notes that when played together, produces a desired sound. Similarly, nutritional harmony describes how the nutrients in whole foods work together to help maintain health. Please note the emphasis on whole foods. There is no one food or magic pill for disease prevention. Rather, it is the balance of whole foods that produces the greatest possible health benefits.

In order to understand how to prevent chronic disease and cancer through nutrition, we must first understand what dietary factors can contribute to the development of chronic disease and cancer. Therefore, the first few chapters are dedicated to understanding how the health of the gastrointestinal tract impacts disease, how food processing diminishes critical nutrients needed for disease prevention, and how specific dietary factors directly contribute to cancer and chronic disease formation. The second half of *Nutritional Harmony* changes focus to illustrate how food can be used to help prevent cancer and chronic disease. These chapters discuss how foods are beneficial and how to select and prepare these foods to optimize their health benefits. Because stress, anxiety, and depression affect all aspects of health, the final chapter discusses the impact of food on stress and mood disorders.

It is beyond the scope of this book to describe all the foods which can impact health. The lists provided are not meant to be comprehensive. Every attempt has been made to provide the most accurate and up to date information. Much of the complicated medical subject matter has been briefly summarized, and a glossary has also been provided to assist the reader with the medical terminology.

Chapter 2

A Healthy Gastrointestinal Tract

Section 1: Leaky Gut

The impact of our diet is not only affected by which foods we choose, but also, the health status of our gastrointestinal tract. Our intestinal barrier is responsible for absorbing what we need (nutrients) and keeping out what we don't need (toxins, bacteria, etc). This barrier is made up of tight cell wall junctions. When there is damage to this barrier, these tight walls weaken, creating gaps in the wall and "leaking." This damage to the intestinal lining can be caused by dysbiosis (an imbalance in the good and bad bacteria), additives/preservatives in our diet, stress and medications. This "leaking" causes inflammation and further damages the lining. As a result, there is a decrease in the absorption of essential vitamins and nutrients (such as the B vitamins and magnesium) and an increase in the absorption of toxins, partially digested foods, and bacteria. The chronic inflammation that results in the body as a result of this "leaking" contributes to most chronic diseases, mood disorders, and cancer growth. Furthermore, as we shall see later, the B vitamins, magnesium, and proper bacterial balance, are all important to cancer and disease prevention.

In addition to the gastrointestinal tract, the liver also serves a critical role in cancer prevention. Liver detoxification rids the body of toxins and carcinogens. Some of the critical nutrients required for this two step process include B vitamins, vitamin E, vitamin C, certain amino acids, glutathione and phytochemicals (the beneficial substances found in plants). When there is an insufficient supply of these nutrients either from a lack of intake or inadequate absorption, the liver's detoxification ability is hindered and therefore, more toxins and carcinogens are absorbed instead of eliminated from the body.

Section 2: Bacterial Balance

The bacteria in the gastrointestinal tract have some of the most important roles in cancer and chronic disease prevention. The balance of good and bad bacteria helps to maintain a healthy intestinal lining (as discussed earlier) and is critical to the proper absorption of nutrients, vitamins, and the elimination of toxins and carcinogens.

There are many factors which can disrupt this balance including specific foods and medications such as antacids, anti-inflammatories and antibiotics. When there is a bacterial infection, antibiotics are essential for destroying the bacteria and restoring health. The antibiotics can also decrease the good bacteria, allowing the bad bacteria to grow and dominate. Many antibiotics are added to animal feed and therefore are present in the meat and dairy products from these animals. This can largely be avoided by consuming organic, grass-fed animal products.

The solution to maintaining the critical bacterial balance lies in feeding the good bacteria and starving the bad bacteria. This can be accomplished by avoiding processed foods and sugar (which feed the bad bacteria) and by increasing our intake of prebiotics (foods that feed the good bacteria). These prebiotic foods include asparagus, garlic, leek, onion, artichoke, banana, oats, soybean, inulin, and dandelion. As we shall see later, many of these prebiotic foods also contain powerful phytochemicals which provide multiple health benefits. There are many sources of these good bacteria including food and probiotic supplements.

Food Sources of Probiotics

- Kefir
- Kombucha tea
- Buttermilk
- Kimchi
- Sauerkraut
- Natto
- Aged cheese-Gouda, Cheddar, Swiss
- Yogurt
- Miso
- Green peas
- Pickles (fermented)
- Probiotic enriched dark chocolate

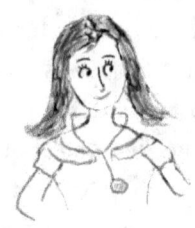 Dark chocolate enriched with probiotics can contain up to four times the amount found in liquid probiotic drinks. One study has found that the bacteria in the enriched dark chocolate are much more likely to survive the passage through the gastrointestinal tract than the bacteria in probiotic enriched milk.[1]

Chapter 3

Nutrients that Impact Chronic Disease

Section 1: The Magic Trio

I often refer to B vitamins, magnesium, and omega-3 fatty acids as a "magic trio" as they impact nearly all chronic disease including mental health, high blood pressure, high cholesterol, diabetes, and cancer. The processing of food contributes to chronic disease by affecting the levels of these critical nutrients. This can best be understood by first reviewing the methods used to process food. A whole grain contains three sections-the bran, endosperm, and germ layers. The bran contains B vitamins, fiber, and the majority of its minerals (such as magnesium, iron, and zinc). The endosperm contains carbohydrates, protein, and only small amounts of vitamins and minerals. The germ layer contains B vitamins, phytonutrients, vitamin E and healthy fats. **When grain is processed the beneficial bran and germ layers are removed, leaving only the endosperm. Thus, the majority of B vitamins, magnesium, and omega-3 fatty acids are lost.** High fructose corn syrup, preservatives/additives, and fat are added to enhance flavor, color, and prolong food's shelf-life. As discussed earlier, these additives contribute to leaky gut and decrease the absorption of vitamins and minerals. **Thus, the processing of foods not only diminishes the amount of these nutrients in food, but also hinders their absorption by damaging the intestinal lining.**

B Vitamins

B vitamins serve many functions in the body including assisting the liver in detoxification and assisting in the formation of neurotransmitters. When the B vitamins are depleted by factors such as processing, stress, caffeine, bacterial imbalance, and certain medications, the liver is less capable of detoxifying the body and therefore, less able to get rid of cancer forming substances. In addition, folate and vitamin B12 are involved in the synthesis of serotonin, the neurotransmitter that affects mood. **Low levels of vitamin B6 have been associated with depression and anxiety.** Some of the common medications which can deplete these critical B vitamins include oral contraceptive pills, diuretics and some diabetic medications. **Several studies have demonstrated that women taking oral contraceptive pills are deficient in vitamin B6 and vitamin B12.**[1] Many foods such as cereals are fortified with B vitamins but other sources include whole grains, nuts, beans, fruits and vegetables. Vitamin B12 is abundant in animal sources such as meat and dairy. For vegans, it can be obtained from vitamin B12 fortified foods.

Omega-3 Fatty Acids

Omega-3 and omega-6 fatty acids are essential fatty acids that must be obtained from our diet as the body is unable to make them. Each of these fatty acids serves a different role in the body. In general, omega-3 fatty acids are anti-inflammatory while omega-6 fatty acids are pro-inflammatory (promote inflammation). The optimum ratio of omega-6:omega-3 fatty acids is 2:1. Due to our current diet, this ratio is much higher, 15-20:1. This reflects a very pro-inflammatory diet which promotes chronic disease as well the growth of cancer.

Our diets are high in omega-6 fatty acids because we consume them directly and indirectly. We consume omega-6 fatty acids directly by consuming oils which are high in omega-6 such as corn oil, sunflower oil, safflower oil, grapeseed oil, and cottonseed oil. We consume them indirectly by consuming animals that have been fed grain. Most animals including cows and chickens are fed a diet of grains usually made with soy or corn. This increases the omega-6 content, causing a higher omega-6:omega-3 ratio. Grass-fed animals provide a much lower omega-6:omega-3 ratio. **In fact, grass-fed animal meat contains nearly five times more omega-3 fatty acids than grain fed meat.** [2] **In addition, grass-fed meat is high in CLA (conjugated linoleic acid). Recent research has demonstrated that CLA may reduce the risk of certain cancers,** but more studies must be done to clarify CLA's potential benefits.[3]

Omega-3 fatty acids improve HTN (high blood pressure), hyperlipidemia (high cholesterol), diabetes, mood disorders, premenstrual syndrome, menopause and inhibit cancer. Optimizing the ratio of omega-6:omega-3 by consuming more omega-3 rich foods is critical to disease prevention.

Common Food Sources of Fatty Acids

Omega-3
Salmon, Sardines, Mackerel
Flaxseed, Chia seeds
Walnuts
Wild rice
Edamame
Omega-3 enriched eggs

CLA
Grass-fed meat
Grass-fed sheep milk>cow milk
Soft cheese>hard cheese

Healthy oils are a good source of omega-3 fatty acids. When cooking with oils, it is important to avoid heating oils above their smoke point. The smoke point is the temperature at which the oil begins to break down altering the flavor of the oil and releasing potentially dangerous compounds. When cooking at high temperatures, consider using an oil with a smoke point of 400 degrees or higher.

- Unrefined safflower, unrefined sunflower, borage, flaxseed and evening primrose oils have low smoke points. They should be added directly to food and not exposed to heat in cooking.

- Different olive oils have different smoke points. **Light refined olive oil has a much higher smoke point (465 degrees fahrenheit) than extra-virgin olive oil (350 degrees fahrenheit).**

- Refined avocado oil has the highest smoke point of 520 degrees.

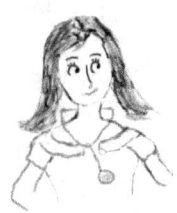 There are many different types of cookware. Aluminum pans can result in aluminum being absorbed into food. Excess aluminum has been linked with Alzheimer's disease, kidney and bone problems. Similarly, the chemical PFOA, used on the surface of many nonstick pans, has been associated with an increased risk of bladder, kidney and testicular cancer in people with large environmental exposures. (No human studies have linked its exposure through cookware to an increased risk of cancer.) If these pans are overheated, they also release gases that cause a flu-like illness. Glass and clay cookware do not cause any chemicals to be released or absorbed into food. Ceramic or porcelain coated cookware is also a good option but is much more expensive. Cast iron cookware is another alternative and allows for some iron to be absorbed from the pan, increasing the iron content of the food being prepared.

Magnesium

Magnesium is an important micronutrient involved in over 300 processes in the body. Magnesium is required for the conversion of vitamin D to its active form and it regulates calcium entry into cells. **It impacts heart disease, migraines, premenstrual syndrome, fibromyalgia, and sleep. Several meta-analyses have demonstrated that the higher the intake of magnesium, the lower the risk of Type 2 diabetes, stroke, and heart disease. In addition, two recent studies have demonstrated an association between a higher intake of magnesium with a lower risk of colon cancer. [4]**

Over 70% of Americans are deficient in this critical nutrient. This is largely due to our current diet and lifestyle. Like B vitamins, magnesium levels are affected by stress and medications such as diuretics and some antacids. Many of the foods we consume also impact magnesium levels. The phosphoric acid in dark soft drinks binds magnesium so that it cannot be used. Artificial saturated fat decreases its absorption while sugar and caffeine cause more magnesium to be excreted by our kidneys.

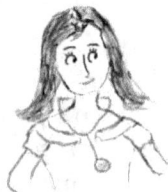

Vitamin B6 helps maintain magnesium levels. Some of the foods rich in both include spinach, wild fish, sesame and pumpkin seeds.

Common Food Sources of Magnesium

Spinach

Swiss chard

Sesame and Pumpkin Seeds

Brazil nuts, Almonds, Cashews

Oat bran

Halibut, Mackerel

Avocado

Dates

Dark Chocolate

Section 2: Vitamin D and K2- The Critical Connection

Vitamin D is a fat-soluble vitamin that is necessary for our bodies to absorb calcium from our diets. It is made in our skin from exposure to sunlight and is present in smaller amounts in certain foods as well as in vitamin D fortified foods. **Vitamin D receptors are present throughout the body. Vitamin D deficiency is associated with nearly all chronic disease states as well as an increased risk of death from all causes.** [5] A recent study demonstrated that people with low vitamin D levels are twice as likely to suffer from depression.[6] Yet another study found that vitamin D levels below 15 were associated with a six-fold increase in the risk of developing high blood pressure in men and a three-fold increase in women.[7] Most recently, a study demonstrated that people over the age of 65 with very low vitamin D levels were over twice as likely to develop Alzheimer's disease and dementia as those with normal levels.[8]

Vitamin D deficiency has been associated with sixteen different cancers. **More than 75% of patients with cancer are vitamin D deficient. Cancer patients with the lowest levels of vitamin D were found to have more advanced cancers at diagnosis.** [9] **Correcting vitamin D deficiency can decrease the overall risk of death from cancer by 29% and decrease the risk of death from breast and colon cancer by 75%.**[10,11] Vitamin D helps kill cancer and is anti-angiogenic (cuts off cancer's blood supply).

In order for vitamin D to work properly, there must be an adequate amount of vitamin K2. Like vitamin D, vitamin K is a fat-soluble vitamin and is found in many foods. Vitamin D is needed for calcium to be absorbed while vitamin K2 guides the calcium to the right place (into the bone where it is needed rather than into our arteries where it contributes to heart disease).

The vitamin K1 form, which is necessary for the proper clotting of our blood, is present in green leafy vegetables. The bacteria in the intestine make a small amount of vitamin K2 from vitamin K1. Recent studies demonstrate that this amount of vitamin K2 is likely not enough and consuming more vitamin K2 rich foods may be needed. A study evaluating heart disease and vitamin K2 consumption found that the **people who consumed the most vitamin K2 were 57% less likely to die from heart disease.**[12] **In a similar study, which followed 24,000 people over a 10 year period, higher vitamin K2 intake was associated with a lower incidence of lung and prostate cancer.** [13] Food sources of vitamin K2 include natto (fermented soy), fermented vegetables, grass-fed dairy products, and some varieties of cheese. Of the cheese sources, Brie and Gouda contain the most vitamin K2.[14]

Chapter 4

Cancer

It is estimated that 70-80% of cancers are due to environmental factors with 30-40% due to diet alone. In order to understand how to prevent cancer through nutrition, we must first have a basic understanding of how cancer forms. Briefly, when the DNA (genetic material) in normal cells become damaged by substances such as carcinogens and free radicals, the cell will usually undergo apoptosis (programmed cell death or cell suicide). Cancer cells are able to avoid this cell death and continue to grow. There are numerous factors in our diet which further promote the growth of cancer cells.

Section 1: Carcinogens

DNA damaging substances that can cause cancer are called carcinogens and include HCAs, nitrosamines, xenoestrogens, and possibly sweeteners, food dyes, and genetically modified foods. **The first step in the dietary prevention of cancer is avoiding the consumption of carcinogens.** It is important to understand the carcinogens in food and how they are formed. The following is a discussion of a few of these carcinogens.

HCAs

Heterocyclic amines are carcinogens that are formed when protein (from animals or fish) is exposed to high temperatures. The higher the temperature and the longer the protein is cooked, the more HCAs form. Therefore, methods of cooking such as barbecuing, charcoal grilling, frying and broiling will lead to the formation of more HCAs than lower temperature methods such as stewing, roasting or boiling. Fortunately, there are ways to minimize the formation of these compounds.

- **Season meat with rosemary, sage, or garlic. One study found that adding rosemary reduced HCA formation by 90%.**[1]

- **Acidic marinades** such as lemon or vinegar based mixtures as well as beer or wine marinades all decrease HCA formation. One study found that marinating meat in a mixture of onion, garlic and lemon juice significantly reduced HCA formation. Of note, the researchers found that the more garlic and onion used in the marinade, the greater the reduction in HCA formation.[2]

- **Microwaving meat** for one to two minutes followed by draining the liquid prior to cooking has been shown to decrease HCA formation by up to 90%.[3] This is likely due to the fact that HCA precursors are water soluble and thus, are lost to the drained fluid. If the meat is cooked with this fluid, the HCA reducing benefit of microwaving is lost.

- Other methods such as **frequently turning meat** while frying and frying in virgin olive oil also reduce HCA formation.[4]

- Meat that is well done has significantly more HCAs than meat that is medium-rare (up to 3.5 times the amount).

- Grilled skinless chicken breast has been shown to contain 100 times more HCAs than a well done hamburger and 17 times more HCAs than a well done steak.[6]

- Consuming green leafy vegetables (such as spinach and kale) which contain chlorophyll has been shown to reduce HCA absorption in the intestine. In one study, high dose chlorophyll blocked HCA absorption by almost 100%.[7]

- Consuming cruciferous vegetables such as broccoli with meat can also block the carcinogenic affects of these HCAs.[8]

PAHs

Polycyclic aromatic hydrocarbons (PAHs) are carcinogens that form when coal, gas, tobacco or other substances are exposed to high heat (charcoal grilling or barbecuing). These substances then bind to the food and have been shown to cause an increased risk of cancer. Smoked foods contain the largest amount of PAHs and have been associated with an increased risk of stomach cancer.[9] Grilling produces the largest amount of PAHs in skinless, boneless chicken breast. Grilled salmon actually contains more PAHs than a well done, grilled hamburger. As with HCAs, studies have demonstrated that an acidic marinade can reduce PAH formation by up to 70%.[10]

Nitrosamines

Nitrosamines are carcinogens found in tobacco from cigarettes and are also formed in nitrite containing foods. Sodium nitrite is used as a preservative in processed meats (hot dogs, sausage, bacon, pepperoni, salami, packaged deli meat). When the nitrite combines with the amino acid in proteins, nitrosamines form. Plants are very high in nitrates which are converted to nitrites by bacteria in the mouth. However, the phytochemicals in plants prevent these plant nitrites from becoming nitrosamines . **This is a critical difference as the consumption of processed meat but not plants is associated with a significantly higher risk of numerous cancers.** The nitrosamine content of one hot dog is alarmingly equivalent to the nitrosamines found in five cigarettes.[11,12]

Multiple studies have demonstrated an increased risk of colon cancer with the consumption of processed meats. **One large study found that men who consumed one ounce of processed meat five to six times a week and women who consumed one ounce two to three times a week had a 50% greater risk of developing colon cancer.**[13] Other studies have also demonstrated a 67% increased risk of pancreatic cancer and a 33% increased risk of bladder cancer.[14,15] **It is useful to note that vitamin C has been shown to block the formation of nitrosamines.** People who consume more vitamin C have lower rates of stomach and colon cancer.[16,17] Some of the vegetables that are highest in vitamin C include peppers and kale. **Kale has thirty times more vitamin C than romaine lettuce and four times the vitamin C in spinach.**

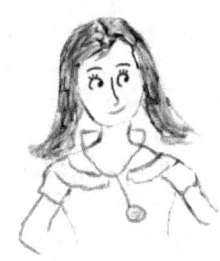 Many "nitrite free" products use celery extract instead of sodium nitrite. Celery is naturally high in nitrites and the phytochemicals in **whole celery** prevent the nitrites from becoming nitrosamines. **Celery extract is an isolated ingredient. We cannot assume that it provides the same protection against nitrosamine formation as the whole food.**

Xenoestrogens

Xenoestrogens are estrogen-like compounds including BPA in plastics, BHA (preservative in food), pesticides, and many other environmental substances. Consumption of dairy and meat from animals treated with hormones also leads to exposure to these compounds. Because these xenoestrogens have estrogen like activity, they can promote the formation of hormone-dependent cancers such as breast, prostate, ovarian, testicular, and endometrial cancers. Many believe that it is this exposure to xenoestrogens through our environment and diet which has led to the rising incidence of hormone-dependent cancers in younger people.

Section 2: The Impact of Sugar

The impact of sugar consumption on cancer formation is controversial. It is well established that obesity itself increases the risk of certain cancers. However, independent of weight, excess sugar promotes inflammation which can lead to chronic disease and cancer (see section 3). When sugar is consumed, insulin levels rise as well as the level of a growth hormone called IGF-1. This is a normal response. However, excess insulin is now thought to be a risk factor for increased tumor growth. Elevated IGF-1 levels have been associated with an increased risk of breast, prostate, and colon cancer.[18] **Most recently, a meta-analysis involving nearly 900,000 participants found that prediabetic patients had a 15% increased risk of developing breast, endometrial, stomach, colorectal, pancreatic and liver cancer. These results were found to be independent of weight.[19]**

The use of artificial sweeteners as an alternative to sugar in some studies, has been associated with weight gain and an increased risk of diabetes. Most recently, a small study conducted on humans found that the consumption of saccharin for just one week altered the bacteria in the intestine. These altered bacteria affected how glucose was metabolized, causing many of the participants' blood sugars to rise to pre-diabetic levels. Similar results were found in mice when they were given saccharin, aspartame or sucralose.[20]

There are many safe alternative sweeteners which may actually have a neutral or positive affect on blood glucose and insulin levels, and thus, avoid the potential cancer risk associated with hyperglycemia. The following is a brief discussion of a few of these sweeteners and how they can contribute to cancer prevention.

Erythritol

Erythritol is a sugar alcohol found naturally in melons and peaches. It provides only one calorie per teaspoon and is 50-70% as sweet as sugar. Recent studies have revealed that erythritol acts as an antioxidant and does not increase blood glucose or insulin levels.[21] In diabetic patients, erythritol has been shown to improve blood vessel function.[22] Erythritol can be purchased in a granular form and can be readily substituted for sugar as it remains stable with heat, making it useful in baking.

Stevia

Stevia is another commonly used natural sweetener. Stevia comes from the Stevia Rebaudiana plant, has zero calories, and is 200-300 times sweeter than regular sugar. The stevia plant contains many phytochemicals and antioxidants and has been shown to have anticancer properties.[23] Studies have found that the use of purified stevia extracts may lower blood pressure as well as blood sugar.[24]

Yacon syrup

Yacon syrup is a molasses-like sweetener made from the root of the Yacon plant. It is made up of 50% FOS (fructooligosacharides) which are indigestible sugars. These fructooligosacharides serve as prebiotics, feeding the good bacteria in the intestine. One study conducted on an elderly population of patients found that the daily consumption of freeze-dried yacon led to a decrease in blood sugar.[25] **In another study, obese premenopausal women given Yacon syrup daily had a notable decrease in fasting insulin levels and significant weight loss but no change in their glucose levels.** [26]

Section 3: Inflammation

Inflammation is a normal response of the immune system that occurs in response to triggers such as infections, toxins, chemicals (such as pesticides), trauma, allergens (such as wheat), and large food particles (as occurs in leaky gut). Normally, once healing occurs, inflammation resolves and does not become chronic. However, if the body continues to be exposed to the trigger, chronic inflammation can occur. This also occurs if the immune system becomes confused and begins to attack normal tissue (which occurs in autoimmune diseases such as lupus and rheumatoid arthritis). The substances released by the immune system that have an effect on other cells are referred to as cytokines. These cytokines can be pro-inflammatory (promoting inflammation) or anti-inflammatory (suppressing inflammation). The presence of inflammation can be determined through blood tests. For example, the CRP (C-reactive protein) is a marker of inflammation and elevated levels have been associated with cancer, diabetes, heart disease, and numerous other conditions.

Other than the common triggers of inflammation, there are many other factors that trigger the release of pro-inflammatory cytokines, promoting chronic inflammation. In obesity, the enlarged adipocytes (fat cells) release these pro-inflammatory cytokines. Sleep deprivation and stress also promote their release.

Diet is the most significant modifiable way to control inflammation. The consumption of sugar, excess omega-6 fatty acids, and artificial trans fats (such as partially hydrogenated oils) found in processed foods is in large part responsible for the chronic inflammation causing chronic disease and cancer.

The explanation of this connection between chronic inflammation, chronic disease and cancer is complicated and continues to be studied. The following is a brief explanation.

Cancer

Chronic inflammation induces changes in cells causing them to release substances that lead to mutations in the DNA and promote the growth of abnormal cells.

Numerous cancers are associated with chronic inflammation and infections such as human papilloma virus and cervical cancer, Hepatitis C and liver cancer, H. Pylori and stomach cancer, inflammatory bowel disease and colon cancer, celiac disease and intestinal lymphoma, and rheumatoid arthritis and lymphoma.

As we have seen in our earlier discussion, obesity causes the release of pro-inflammatory cytokines. Obesity is associated with an increased risk of breast, esophageal, liver, colon, and endometrial cancer.

Diabetes

Pro-inflammatory cytokines have been shown to affect the cell's response to insulin, causing insulin resistance (diabetes). An elevated CRP (a marker of inflammation) has been shown to be predictive of diabetes before it is diagnosed. One study found that women with high CRP levels were eight times more likely to develop diabetes while men with high CRP levels were twice as likely to develop diabetes than those with normal levels.[27]

Heart disease and Stroke

When blood vessels are damaged (by smoking, diabetes, or high blood pressure), cholesterol becomes deposited. Chronic inflammation can cause these cholesterol deposits or plaques to become unstable. When a piece of this unstable plaque breaks off a stroke or heart attack can occur. A dislodged plaque in the coronary arteries of the heart causes a heart attack while in the arteries leading to the brain causes a stroke. An elevated CRP has been shown to be a greater predictor for the risk of a heart attack or stroke than the LDL ("bad") cholesterol.[28]

Exercise and Inflammation

The value of exercise for the prevention of heart disease, mood disorders and neurodegenerative diseases is well established. Exercise also has a protective role in decreasing the risk of lung, breast, endometrial, colon, prostate, and kidney cancers. It can also decrease the side effects of cancer treatment and decrease cancer related mortality. One of the main ways that moderate exercise impacts disease is by decreasing inflammation as demonstrated by lower CRP levels.

Chapter 5

Food as Medicine

Cancer Prevention

The impact of food on cancer formation, growth, and metastasis (spread) cannot be underestimated. In a review of 200 studies, it was found that **those people who consume the least amount of fruits and vegetables have twice the risk of developing cancer as those who consume the most fruits and vegetables.**[1] In order to have a better understanding of why specific foods improve health, many of the following sections highlight specific phytochemicals found in these foods. However, once again, **it is the harmony of the all the nutrients in the whole food which provides the greatest benefit.**

The impact of diet on prostate and breast cancer, the leading causes of cancer among men and women, has been extensively studied.

Prostate Cancer

Prostate cancer is the most common cancer in men and the second leading cause of cancer death.

In 2005, a study was conducted on 93 men with early stage prostate cancer who elected not to have surgery but simply monitor their PSA. The PSA is a blood test that is used to monitor prostate cancer. The men were split into two groups. One group adopted a vegetarian diet with supplements, exercised six days per week, and participated in stress management as well as a weekly support group. The other group made no changes. The group that implemented changes had an improvement in their PSA while the group that made no changes had a rise (worsening) in their PSA with some requiring chemotherapy, surgery, and radiation.[2]

In the Harvard Physicians Health Study, involving over 20,000 male physicians, men who consumed more than 600mg of calcium (two or more servings per day) from dairy had a 32% greater risk of developing prostate cancer.[3] For prostate cancer prevention, one study involving 47,000 male participants found that **those men who consumed ten or more servings of tomatoes per week lowered their risk of prostate cancer by 45%.**[4] In patients who already have prostate cancer, **pomegranate juice and flaxseed have also been shown to slow the growth of prostate cancer.** [5,6]

Breast Cancer

Breast cancer is the leading cause of cancer in women and the second leading cause of cancer death. Numerous studies have evaluated the impact of food on breast cancer.

A large study involving 88,803 premenopausal women found that **those women who consumed the most red meat had a 22% increased risk of developing breast cancer. Every additional serving of red meat per day led to a 13% increase in breast cancer risk. Substituting one serving of red meat for one serving of legumes, decreased the risk by 15%.**[7] In another study conducted on 93,676 postmenopausal women, the incidence of breast cancer in women with the highest insulin levels was 2.4 times higher than those women with the lowest insulin levels.[8] **Other nutritional factors associated with an increased risk of breast cancer include alcohol use, vitamin D deficiency, and selenium deficiency.**

As we shall see in this chapter, there are many foods that can help prevent breast cancer. Multiple studies have demonstrated that women who consume more cruciferous vegetables have a lower risk of breast cancer.[9] Women with higher levels of B vitamins, magnesium and omega-3 fatty acids (the "magic trio") also have a lower incidence of breast cancer.[10,11,12] **In a study conducted on women who carried the breast cancer gene (in whom their risk of developing breast cancer is 80%), those women who consumed several servings of a variety of fruits and vegetables a day had a significant decrease in their risk of developing breast cancer even though they carried the breast cancer gene.** [13]

The survival of women who have breast cancer is also impacted by their diet and lifestyle. In one study, women with breast cancer who consumed 5 fruits and vegetables daily and exercised 30 minutes per day, six days per week, had a 50% lower risk of death than those who did not make these changes.[14]

"Let food be thy medicine and medicine be thy food"

-Hippocrates

Section 1: Vegetables

The Alliums

The allium vegetables include garlic, onions, scallions, chives, and leeks. Their antioxidant and anti-inflammatory activities provide numerous health benefits. Many of the allium vegetables have been shown to help prevent and treat heart disease and diabetes. **Garlic is the most effective vegetable against nearly every form of cancer.** In a recent in vitro study comparing the most effective cancer fighting vegetables, garlic was most effective against breast, brain, lung, pancreatic, prostate and stomach cancers.[1] Allicin, the anticancer phytochemical in garlic, is not present in garlic but is created from garlic. Whole garlic contains the two substances (allin and the enzyme that acts upon it, allinase) which are needed to form allicin. These two substances combine only when garlic is processed (by chopping, pressing, crushing, etc). After processing, it is critical to allow the garlic to rest for ten minutes prior to exposing it to heat. If the processed garlic is immediately exposed to heat, the enzyme responsible for forming allicin becomes inactivated and no allicin will form. Similarly, acidic foods such as lemon juice also deactivate the enzyme and should not be immediately added to freshly cut garlic until it has been allowed to rest for five to ten minutes.

In a study comparing other allium vegetables, shallots had the highest antioxidant activity followed by Western Yellow, New York Bold, and Northern Red onions.[2] One of the principal anticancer phytochemicals in shallots and onions is **quercetin.** Quercetin has also been shown to lower blood pressure, improve mood, and acts as a natural antihistamine.[3]

Of the alliums, shallots have the highest content of quercetin followed by onions. Yellow and red onions have more quercetin than white onions.[4] When selecting onions, consider choosing organic onions as conventional onions have usually been irradiated and have a lower quercetin concentration. Peel onions minimally as the concentration of quercetin is higher in the outer layers of the onion.[5] **Unlike many vegetables, cooking onions in any way (except for boiling) improves their anticancer benefits by improving quercetin's bioavailability** (**the amount absorbed**). [6] Of note, capers, which are not members of the allium family, have the highest quercetin content of any food (nearly seven times the amount found in red onions).[7]

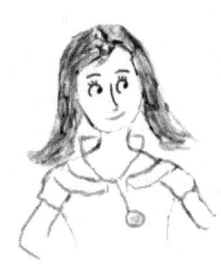 A recent study demonstrated that sprouted garlic which has green shoots stemming from the cloves has much more antioxidant activity than fresh garlic. In fact, the garlic that sprouted for five days had the highest antioxidant activity when compared to fresh garlic or garlic sprouted for less than five days.[8]

Cruciferous Vegetables

The harmony among the phytochemicals, vitamins, minerals, fiber and omega-3 fatty acids in crucifers is responsible for their extensive health benefits. Some of the most common crucifers include broccoli, cauliflower, kale, watercress, brussels sprouts, and cabbage. Crucifers contain magnesium, B vitamins, omega-3 fatty acids (the "magic trio"), and vitamin K all of which impact chronic disease and cancer. They are also very high in carotenoids and vitamin C, giving them powerful antioxidant properties. Carotenoids are the yellow, orange, and red pigments in crucifers and other fruits and vegetables. As we shall see later, two of these carotenoids, beta-carotene and lycopene, have been extensively studied for their health benefits.

The phytochemicals in cruciferous vegetables help prevent normal cells from becoming abnormal, help rid the body of carcinogens before DNA damage occurs, slow cancer cell growth, induce apoptosis (cancer cell death), and block angiogenesis (thereby depriving the cancer of its blood supply and nutrients it needs to grow). Consuming cruciferous vegetables has been shown to reduce the risk of developing many different types of cancers.

- **One study found a 50% reduction in the risk of breast cancer simply when the participants consumed one cruciferous vegetable per day.[1]**

- **Another study found that men who consumed only three servings a week, had a 41% reduction in the risk of prostate cancer.[2]**

Cruciferous vegetables have also been shown to benefit the heart with one study demonstrating that a high cruciferous vegetable intake was associated with a decrease in the risk of death from heart disease.[3] They contain varying amounts of the phytochemical glucosinolate and the enzyme myrosinase. Similar to garlic, their main anticancer phytochemicals (isothiocyanates and indoles) are not present in the cruciferous vegetables but rather, are released from the vegetables when myrosinase acts on the glucosinolates present in the vegetables.

Once again, proper selection and preparation are key to maximizing the anticancer properties of these vegetables. In order to form these anticancer phytochemicals, the myrosinase enzyme must be activated by either cutting the broccoli or by adding a vitamin C rich food (such as lemon juice). Myrosinase is inactivated by heat. Therefore, it is best to consume raw crucifers which have been cut and then allowed to rest for five minutes, giving the myrosinase sufficient time to work. When cooking crucifers, it is best to lightly steam them for less than five minutes, using the least amount of water as their phytochemicals are water soluble.

Cruciferous Vegetables in order of Glucosinolate Content[4]

Brussels sprouts- contain the most

Broccoli sprouts- contain nearly four times the amount in broccoli

Cress

Mustard greens

Kale- curly kale contains more than Chinese kale

Broccoli

Cabbage- Chinese cabbage has less than white, red or savoy varieties

---

Carrots

As with many vegetables, carrots provide many anticancer phytochemicals, vitamins and fiber. The rich color of carrots comes from the carotenoid, beta-carotene. Beta-carotene acts as an antioxidant and is converted to vitamin A in the intestine. Carrots also contain the natural anti-fungal compound, falcarinol. In animal studies, falcarinol has been shown to reduce the risk of developing colon cancer.[1] Other studies have demonstrated that carrot consumption can reduce the risk of heart disease by up to 32%.[2] A recent study comparing the falcarinol content of carrot varieties found that **deep purple carrots contain the highest concentration of falcarinol** when compared to orange, white and red varieties.[3]

Cooking methods affect the level of these phytonutrients in different ways. **Boiling improves the bioavailability of carotenoids and therefore increases the amount of carotenoids absorbed, but significantly decreases the amount of falcarinol in the carrots.**[4] Because carotenoids are fat soluble, consuming carrots with a healthy fat such as olive oil improves the amount of carotenoids absorbed.

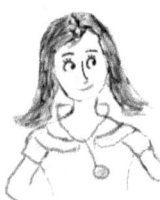

Be sure to cut the green tops off of carrots, beets, and radishes before refrigerating them. The greens draw moisture from the root, causing them to dry out or wilt more quickly.

Spinach

Spinach is an excellent source of magnesium, potassium, many of the B vitamins, vitamin K, and vitamin A. Similar to carrots, cooking spinach improves the bioavailability of its beta-carotene. **Raw spinach's beta-carotene bioavailability is also influenced by how it is processed such that liquefied spinach contains more bioavailable beta-carotene than minced or whole spinach.**[1] **Liquefied and minced spinach also have more bioavailable folate than whole spinach.** [2] Therefore, if choosing to consume fresh spinach, consider mincing it, juicing it or adding it to a smoothie to maximize its nutritional value.

- Raw spinach is high in oxalic acid which interferes with the absorption of the calcium in spinach. Cooking spinach breaks down this oxalic acid, improving calcium absorption.

- Spinach also contains lutein and zeaxanthin which make up part of the retina of the eye. Studies have demonstrated that foods high in these two carotenoids may help prevent age related macular degeneration as well as cataracts.[3]

A recent study evaluated the effects of light exposure on spinach. The researchers placed spinach in containers similar to the clear containers found in grocery stores and then exposed one group to light which was also similar to the lighting found in grocery stores. The second group of spinach containers was placed in the dark. **They found that the spinach exposed to the light increased in nutritional value (higher vitamin content) while that exposed to the dark had a decrease in the level of some of the vitamins.** [4]

Section 2: Fruits

Like vegetables, the nutritional harmony created in fruit provides greater health benefits than supplementing with any one component. In addition to their high antioxidant content and anti-inflammatory properties, fruits contain fiber and numerous anticancer phytochemicals. They can help regulate blood sugar, lower blood pressure, lower cholesterol, prevent age related diseases (such as Alzheimer's disease), and help prevent cancer. A recent in vitro study comparing fruits found that **cranberries and lemons decreased cancer cell proliferation the most followed by apples, strawberries, and red grapes.** The same study also found that antioxidant activity was highest in cranberries followed by apples, red grapes, strawberries, peaches, lemons, pears, bananas, oranges, grapefruits, and pineapples.[1] Much of the anticancer benefit of these fruits lies in their skin or peel.

In fact, one study demonstrated that simply consuming one tablespoon of citrus zest per week led to a 34% reduction in the risk of skin cancer.[2] When consuming the peel or skin of fruits and vegetables, it is important to minimize exposure to pesticides by choosing organic produce.

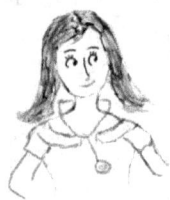

To clean fruit, combine one part white distilled vinegar to three parts water in a spray bottle, shake, spray the fruit, let rest for thirty seconds, rub gently, then rinse with cold water.

Apples

The apple's numerous health benefits include lowering cholesterol, stabilizing blood sugar, and reducing the risk of cancers such as breast, prostate, and many others.[1] One study found that women who consumed 3 ounces of dried apple rings daily for one year had a 23% drop in their LDL.[2] A study comparing twenty-one varieties of apples found that of the common apples consumed, **Idared apples are the healthiest** followed by Red Delicious, Honeycrisp, and Granny Smith. In this study, Golden Nugget apples were found to be the least nutritious.[3]

The apple's peel contains a much higher concentration of phytochemicals (such as quercetin) than the flesh. Surprisingly, freeze dried apple peels have a higher concentration of phytochemicals than fresh apple peels. If choosing to consume the apple peels, consider choosing organic apples to avoid the pesticides on the skin of conventional apples. Unlike apple peels, apple juice and sauce have a much lower phytochemical concentration.[4]

Citrus Fruits

The health benefits of citrus fruits extend far beyond their high concentration of vitamin C. Citrus fruits contain many phytochemicals (such as hesperidin, limonoids, and naringin) with antioxidant, anticancer, and anti-inflammatory properties. Studies have found that women with the highest citrus intake had at least a 10% reduced risk of breast cancer as well as a reduced risk of heart disease and stroke.[1,2,3]

Oranges contain the most hesperidin, an anticancer phytochemical which inhibits breast and prostate cancer cells in vitro.[4] Of the orange varieties, **clementines contain the highest concentration of hesperidin** while navel oranges contain the least.[5] Navel orange peels also contain half of the limonoids found in Valencia oranges.[6]

Grapefruit peels contain the highest concentration of limonoids. However, the main anticancer phytochemical found in grapefruit is naringin, a phytochemical which, in vitro, has been shown to inhibit numerous cancers including breast, colon, lung, and skin cancer.[7] Of note, **white grapefruit contains much higher concentrations of naringin than pink or red varieties.**[8]

Berries

Anthocyanins are the phytochemicals that give berries their rich color. These anthocyanins have anti-inflammatory, antioxidant, and anticancer effects and help prevent heart disease, cancer, and neurodegenerative diseases. In a study comparing the anthocyanin content of fruits and vegetables, chokeberries and elderberries contained the very highest concentrations (1480mg/ 100g and 1375mg/ 100g respectively). Black raspberries (687mg/ 100g), wild blueberries (487mg/ 100g), blackberries (300mg/ 100g), black plums (124.5mg/ 100 grams), and concord grapes (120mg/ 100g) also contain very high concentrations. Vegetables were also evaluated in this study with red cabbage, red radishes, and eggplants found to be superior in anthocyanin content to black beans, red beans, and red onions.[1]

Ellagic acid is also found in berries and has been shown to impact cancer at multiple levels by preventing carcinogens from damaging DNA, stopping cancer growth as well as cutting off cancer's blood supply (anti-angiogenesis). In a human study conducted on colon cancer patients before surgery, the consumption of black raspberry powder not only decreased the growth rate of the tumors but also caused death of the tumor cells.[2] **Red raspberries and blackberries contain the highest concentration of ellagic acid.** Strawberries, cranberries and pomegranates also contain ellagic acid but in lower concentrations.[3]

In addition to the well documented anticancer and anti-inflammatory effects of berries, there are numerous studies which demonstrate that berries can help prevent diabetes. For example, in a study conducted on overweight healthy adults, one month of **acai pulp** (100 grams twice daily) led to a reduction in fasting glucose, insulin, and cholesterol levels.[4] Similarly, a study conducted on Type 2 diabetics demonstrated that **bilberry** extract reduced post-prandial blood sugar (the blood sugar level after eating) and insulin levels.[5] Yet another study conducted on both diabetic and non-diabetic patients found that consuming **Amla** (Indian gooseberry) extract for 21 days significantly lowered blood sugar and cholesterol in both groups.[6]

There are many factors to consider when purchasing and preparing berries. It is advisable to purchase organic berries whenever possible. Frozen berries (especially flash frozen berries) are almost as nutritious as fresh berries. Consider quickly thawing berries in the microwave. One study found that thawing strawberries in the microwave maintained more antioxidants than thawing them at room temperature.[7] Freeze-dried berries are a good alternative to fresh berries as they retain their anthocyanin content.[8] The ellagitannins (precursors to ellagic acid) in berries remain stable with freezing, canning, pureeing, or heating. However, the removal of seeds when juicing diminishes the ellagitannin content as the seeds contain a high concentration of ellagitannin.[9] When selecting cranberry juice, consider choosing the juice which is not from concentrate as it contains nearly twice the anthocyanins found in the juice from concentrate. Homemade cranberry sauce has 40% more anthocyanins than canned sauce made from whole cranberries and 93% more than canned cranberry jelly.[10]

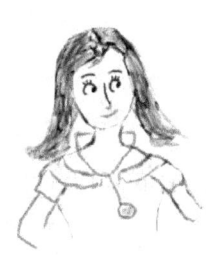

Tart cherries are one of the most effective anti-inflammatory foods. The anthocyanins in tart cherries have been shown to significantly improve pain in people with osteoarthritis and have also been shown to prevent gout attacks. Because tart cherries are naturally high in melatonin, tart cherry juice can be a very beneficial sleep aid.

Tomatoes

Lycopene is one of the anticancer phytochemicals found in tomatoes, watermelon, guava, pink grapefruit, and papaya. Of note, one wedge of watermelon contains four times the lycopene content of one tomato.[1] Seedless watermelon contains more lycopene than watermelon containing seeds.[2] Cherry tomatoes have a much higher lycopene content than cluster or round tomatoes.[3] When cooking with tomatoes, it is important to utilize the skin as it contains up to five times more lycopene than the pulp.[4] The amount of bioavailable lycopene increases when tomatoes are cooked. In fact, cooking tomatoes for thirty minutes has been shown to double the amount of lycopene absorbed.[5] This explains why two tablespoons of tomato paste contains three times the lycopene found in one medium raw tomato.[1] Because lycopene is fat-soluble, it is important to consume or cook tomatoes with a healthy fat such as olive oil or avocados. Also, consider choosing organic tomatoes as they have a much higher lycopene content than conventional tomatoes.

Avocados

Avocados are considered fruit and are an excellent source of fiber, magnesium, vitamin E, vitamin C, vitamin K1, and many of the B vitamins. Phytosterols in avocados are plant cholesterols that help prevent the absorption of "bad" cholesterol from other foods. The carotenoids in avocados have demonstrated anticancer benefits. In vitro studies found that avocado extract stopped the growth of prostate and oral cancer cells. **The highest concentration of avocados' anticancer carotenoids is found closest to the avocado peel.** [1] Therefore, when preparing avocados, it is best to peel the skin off of avocados in order to retain as much of the fruit that is closest to the peel. In addition, the good fats found in avocados improve the carotenoid and lycopene absorption from other vegetables.

Most avocados in the United States are grown in California or Florida. Of the numerous varieties available, the Haas and Fuerte varieties are the most common. The Haas avocado is available year round and its thick skin darkens as it becomes ripe. The Fuerte avocado is available from late fall to the spring and its skin remains green as it becomes ripe. **The Haas avocado contains more anticancer carotenoids than the Fuerte.**[1]

Section 3: Legumes

Legumes include beans, lentils, peanuts, peas, and soybeans. Legumes are high in protein, fiber, minerals, and the "magic trio" of magnesium, omega-3 fatty acids, and B vitamins. The anticancer benefit of legumes includes their high antioxidant and fiber content as well as numerous anticancer phytochemicals. Women who consume beans or lentils two or more times per week have a 24% lower risk of developing breast cancer.[1] **In a study conducted on people over the age of 70, there was an 8% reduced risk of death for every 20 grams of beans (slightly more than one tablespoon) consumed per day.** [2] Cooked and canned beans have nearly the same nutritional value, but canned beans can be very high in sodium. This excess sodium can be avoided by purchasing the "no added salt" varieties.

The consumption of soy products has increased significantly. The controversy surrounding the health benefits of soy consumption is related to the activity of its phytochemical isoflavones (genistein and daidzein). **Miso has more isoflavones than edamame followed by dry roasted soybeans.** These isoflavones have been shown to stop tumor growth and to be anti-angiogenic but are controversial because of their weak estrogen-like activity. Studies have demonstrated mixed results with some demonstrating a decreased risk of breast cancer particularly when soy is consumed prior to puberty or in adolescence. Other human studies have shown no association while some animal studies demonstrated an increase in risk. In human studies, the use of processed soy in the form of supplements has been shown to be associated with an increased risk of breast cancer. There-fore, because of the significant amount of contradictory information surrounding the use of soy, the following is advisable.

- Always consult with your medical provider es-pecially if you have cancer, a family history of hormone-dependent cancer, if you are meno-pausal, or post-menopausal.

- Avoid processed soy products.

- Purchase organic, non-GMO soy products.

- Whole soy foods (edamame or dry roasted soy-beans) and fermented soy foods (such as miso, natto, or tempeh) are healthier than processed soy products.

Section 4: Nuts

Nuts have consistently demonstrated health benefits for cancer prevention, heart disease, diabetes and mood disorders. Nuts are not only an excellent source of the "magic trio" (omega-3 fatty acids, magnesium, B vita-mins) but are also high in vitamin E, protein, and fiber. **Compared to other common nuts, almonds and pista-chios provide the most protein and fiber while almonds and pecans provide the most vitamin E.**[1] Nuts are also high in the amino acid arginine. Butternuts (similar to walnuts) have more arginine than any other nut fol-lowed by black walnuts and almonds.[2] In the body, ar-ginine is converted to nitrous oxide which relaxes blood vessels (thereby lowering blood pressure) and improves bloodflow. Nuts also help prevent heart disease by improving cholesterol (decreasing LDL and raising HDL) as well as decreasing inflammation. Studies have shown that women who consume five ounces of nuts per week have a 35% lower risk of heart disease while men who eat nuts twice a week decrease their risk of sudden cardiac death by 47%.[3,4] **In a large study with over 100,000 participants, consumption of one ounce of nuts per day was associated with a 20% lower risk of death from heart disease or cancer.**[5] Yet another study found that the consumption of one ounce of nuts five or more times per week was associated with a 27% decrease in the risk of developing Type 2 diabetes.[6] Although nuts are high in calories, studies have shown that people who consume nuts twice a week are much less likely to gain weight than those people who rarely consume nuts.[7]

Walnuts

- Walnuts are **higher in antioxidants** than any other nut and have been shown in test tube studies to decrease cancer cell growth more than any other nut. (Pecans are second to walnuts in anti-cancer activity and antioxidant content).[1]

- English walnuts are much higher in antioxidants than black walnuts but are much lower in arginine.[2]

- Consume both the walnut and its bitter skin as the skin contains 90% of its antioxidant content.[3] Walnuts have been shown to directly impact the genes responsible for breast cancer development. Animal studies have demonstrated that consuming the equivalent of two ounces per day can cut the risk of breast cancer in half while consuming three ounces per day can lead to a 50% decrease in the size of prostate tumors.[4,5,6]

- ALA which is the main omega-3 fatty acid in walnuts has been shown to impact brain function, improving memory and helping to prevent dementia.

Almonds

- Almonds contain more **calcium** than any other nut. They are also high in magnesium. As we know from our earlier discussion, magnesium, vitamin D, and vitamin K2 all work together for the proper absorption and distribution of calcium into the bone. In fact, the consumption of almonds has been shown to improve bone density by decreasing the formation of osteoclasts (the cells that breakdown and resorb bone).[1]

Pistachios

- Potassium rich foods can help lower blood pressure and pistachios contain more **potassium** per serving than any other nut.[1]

- Pistachios contain more phytosterols (plant cholesterols) than any other nut and thus, can significantly lower cholesterol.[2]

- In a recent study conducted on men with erectile dysfunction, the consumption of 100 grams (roughly 3 ounces) of pistachios per day for three weeks led to an improvement in erections. This improvement was reported by participants as well as documented by ultrasound which revealed increased blood flow.[3]

Brazil nuts

- One Brazil nut contains more than 100% of the RDA of **selenium**. Selenium is necessary for proper thyroid function and has also been shown to help prevent cancer. In a large review of selenium and cancer, those people who consumed the most selenium in their diets had a 31% lower risk of cancer than those who consumed the least amount of selenium in their diets.[1] Brazil nuts also contain more magnesium than other nuts followed by cashews then almonds.

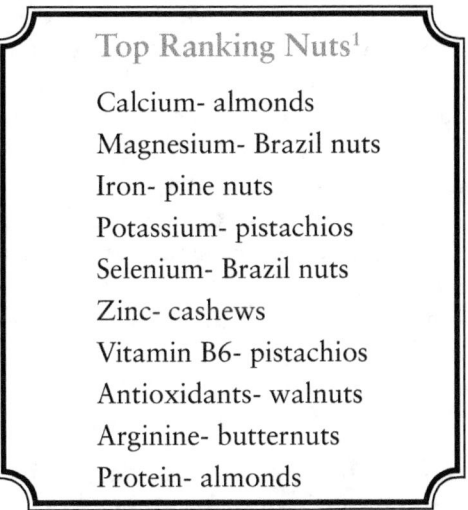

Top Ranking Nuts[1]

Calcium- almonds

Magnesium- Brazil nuts

Iron- pine nuts

Potassium- pistachios

Selenium- Brazil nuts

Zinc- cashews

Vitamin B6- pistachios

Antioxidants- walnuts

Arginine- butternuts

Protein- almonds

Section 5: Seeds

Seeds are high in the "magic trio" and thus, may help prevent chronic disease and cancer. Of all the seeds, **pumpkin seeds have the highest magnesium content** followed by sesame and sunflower seeds. As we shall see later, these three seeds are also high in tryptophan and thus, have a positive impact on mood by increasing serotonin levels. Pumpkin and sesame seeds are also high in zinc which is necessary for the formation of serotonin and GABA (two of the main neurotransmitters responsible for mood).

Flaxseeds

Flaxseeds have well established antioxidant and anti-inflammatory benefits. They are rich in fiber, contain the highest concentration of ALA (an omega-3 fatty acid) and plant lignans. These lignans are phytoestrogens (plants with estrogen-like activity) and have been shown to help prevent breast, prostate and colon cancer.[1,2,3] To maximize the nutritional value of flaxseed consume ground flaxseed instead of whole flaxseed. Once ground, it should be stored in a dark, air-tight container in the refrigerator. This allows it to last up to 3 months. Flaxseed oil contains ALA but does not provide the fiber or lignans that the whole or ground flaxseed provides. In addition, flaxseed oil has a low smoke point and therefore should not be exposed to heat in cooking.

Chia Seeds

Chia seeds come from the plant Salvia hispanica. Unlike flaxseed, chia seeds do not have to be ground to obtain their health benefits. However, one study comparing ground to whole chia found that those participants who consumed ground chia had an increase in their omega-3 fatty acid levels (a 58% increase in their EPA levels and a 39% increase in their ALA levels). Those who consumed whole chia had no increase in these omega-3 levels.[1] When compared to flaxseed, ounce for ounce, chia seeds are higher in antioxidants and provide more fiber, calcium, and iron than flaxseed. However, flaxseed is much higher in anticancer lignans and also contains more omega-3 fatty acids, magnesium, phosphorus and potassium.

Section 6: Mushrooms

White button, shiitake, maitake, and reishi mushrooms have demonstrated significant anticancer properties. **It is important to cook all mushrooms prior to consuming as many mushrooms including the Agaricus bisporus (white, cremini, and portobello) mushrooms and Lentinula erodes (shiitake) mushrooms contain the carcinogen agaritine.** The most effective way to destroy agaritine is by microwaving, frying or boiling the mushrooms while dry baking is the least effective way of destroying agaritine.[1] White button mushrooms have been shown to be very effective against breast cancer. In fact, in a study done on Chinese women, those women who consumed an average of 10 grams, approximately one, white button mushroom per day, had a 64% decreased risk of developing breast cancer.[2] Shiitake mushrooms contain the phytochemical lentinan which in Japan, is given to gastric cancer patients intravenously and has been shown to prolong survival in patients with advanced disease.[3]

Section 7: Green Tea

Green tea has been shown to affect nearly all chronic disease including heart disease (lowering cholesterol and coronary artery disease), diabetes, stroke, mood disorders, and cancer. In a large study conducted over

11 years, **the risk of death from all causes was 23% lower in women who drank five or more cups per day and 12% lower in men.**[1] Catechins are the anticancer phytochemical in tea. EGCG is the main catechin in green tea responsible for most of its health benefits. In a 15 year study conducted with 61,000 women ages 40-76 with no history of cancer, there was a 24% reduction in the risk of ovarian cancer with one cup of green tea and a 46% reduction with 2 cups.[2] Other studies have demonstrated that green tea consumption is associated with a 22% reduced risk of developing breast cancer, a 48% reduced risk of prostate cancer, and a 57% reduced risk of colorectal cancer.[3,4,5]

Green tea has the highest catechin content of all the varieties of teas. Loose green tea is higher in catechins than tea in bags. It is best to use the tea within six months as tea catechins begin to break down after 6 months.

When preparing green tea, it should be steeped for at least 5-8 minutes. Placing lemon juice in the cup or pot prior to brewing will significantly increase the amount of cancer fighting EGCG absorbed.

Section 8: Herbs and Spices

There are many herbs and spices which provide anticancer phytochemicals. Parsley, rosemary, turmeric, allspice, basil, caraway, cardamom, cinnamon, clove, coriander, cumin, dill, and ginger have all been studied for their health and anticancer benefits. Below is a brief description of a few of these herbs.

Parsley

Parsley is an excellent source of vitamins C, K, betacarotene, iron and folate. It has powerful antioxidant and anti-inflammatory properties.

- **Myristicin is the oil in parsley which has been shown to neutralize one of the cancer forming compounds formed during charcoal grilling.[1]**

- In animal and in vitro studies, parsley's phytochemical **apigenin** has been shown to impact many different types of cancer including leukemia, breast, prostate, ovarian, and cervical cancer. **One human study comparing women's dietary intakes found that women with the highest apigenin intake had a 28% lower risk of ovarian cancer.[2]**

- Dried parsley contains significantly higher concentrations of apigenin than fresh parsley. Other herbs such as peppermint, and thyme also contain apigenin.

Rosemary

- Rosemary contains the phytochemicals carnosic acid and rosmarinic acid both of which in vitro, have demonstrated anticancer activity against leukemia, breast, prostate, liver, and lung cancer.[1]

- As we saw in our earlier discussion of carcinogens, rosemary can block the formation of the HCAs that form in animal products when they are cooked at high temperatures. **In fact, rosemary is the most effective herb at blocking HCA formation.**

Turmeric

Turmeric is one of the most powerful spices for cancer and chronic disease prevention with thousands of studies demonstrating its large range of effects. Curcumin is the active ingredient in turmeric responsible for its anti-cancer, anti-inflammatory and antioxidant effects. Adding black pepper to turmeric increases the absorption of its curcumin by nearly 2000%. Of note, because of its poor bioavailability, most studies have been conducted with turmeric curcumin supplements.

Curcumin crosses the blood brain barrier and exerts many positive effects. For example, it increases the amount of BDNF, a growth factor in the brain. BDNF is responsible for the formation of new neurons (brain cells). Therefore, by increasing the concentration of BDNF, **turmeric curcumin promotes the formation of new neurons in the brain.** Exercise, DHA (an omega-3 fatty acid), and caloric restriction can also increase BDNF levels. Turmeric may also help prevent and treat Alzheimer's disease. It has been shown to help prevent the formation of beta amyloid plaques which are found in the brain of Alzheimer's patients.[1,2] Turmeric may also improve depression. One study found that in patients with MDD (major depressive disorder) taking one gram of curcumin was as effective in treating depression as prescription anti-depressant medication.[3] In animal studies, it has also been shown to increase levels of serotonin (the neurotransmitter that affects mood).[4]

Other studies have demonstrated that **turmeric curcumin helps to prevent heart disease.** The blood vessels in the body have a lining of cells called endothelial cells that make up this lining. If this lining is not functioning properly, known as endothelial dysfunction, high blood pressure and coronary artery disease (blocked arteries) can occur. Turmeric has been shown to improve this endothelial function.[5] Turmeric has also been shown to prevent LDL oxidation. (Oxidized LDL is the type of cholesterol that contributes to blockage in the arteries.)[6]

As we have seen, chronic inflammation is the root cause of most chronic disease and contributes to cancer formation. **Turmeric curcumin is a potent anti-inflammatory.** In patients with rheumatoid arthritis, it has been shown to be more effective in improving symptoms than prescription anti-inflammatory medications.[7] It has also been shown to be beneficial in the treatment of other autoimmune diseases such as psoriasis, scleroderma, lupus, and inflammatory bowel disease. Other studies have found it to be as effective as prescription anti-inflammatory medications for conditions such as osteoarthritis but without the same toxicity that is often associated with prescription anti-inflammatory medications.

In diabetic mice, curcumin has been shown to decrease blood sugar levels,[8] and numerous animal studies have found that it helps to prevent the complications associated with diabetes such as kidney disease, retinopathy (damage to the retina), cardiomyopathy (enlargement of the heart), and neuropathy (damage to the nerves).

Turmeric impacts cancer at all stages of cancer development. It prevents cancer formation, stops cancer growth, and prevents the spread of cancer (referred to as metastasis). In vitro studies have found curcumin to prevent the growth of breast, head and neck, liver, pancreatic, colon, prostate, ovarian, brain, blood and skin cancers.[9,10]

Section 9: Food Synergy

Just as the individual components in whole foods work together in harmony, the combination of whole foods together has also been shown to have added health benefits. Food synergy occurs when a combination of foods together produces a greater result than the sum of their individual results.

There are many studies demonstrating the synergy of cruciferous vegetables with other foods. For example, in animal studies, feeding rats the combination of broccoli and tomatoes was much more effective in reducing prostate cancer tumor size than either broccoli or tomatoes alone. It is interesting to note that when these rats were fed only lycopene (the main carotenoid in tomatoes) there was an insignificant decrease in the size of the tumor while feeding the rats whole tomatoes reduced tumor size by 34%.[1] This further demonstrates how the nutritional harmony created in whole foods provides more health benefits than the isolated components of these foods.

The synergy between tea and many foods has been consistently demonstrated in both animal and human studies. For example, as we have already seen, both green tea and mushroom consumption have been shown to decrease the risk of breast cancer. In the same mushroom study, women who consumed an average of one white button mushroom per day and drank one or more grams of steeped green tea a day had an additional 25% reduction in their risk of breast cancer.[2] In animal studies conducted on mice with sarcoma (a cancer of the muscles), the combination of reishi mushroom and green tea extract inhibited the growth of the sarcoma and prolonged survival.[3]

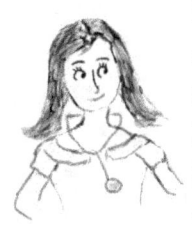

It is also important to note that food combinations can impact the absorption of their nutrients and vitamins. For example, consuming foods high in vitamin C and iron improves the absorption of iron. However, consuming certain teas (black, green, and oolong) with iron-rich vegetables can actually prevent the absorption of non-heme iron.

Chapter 6

Harmony of the Mind

As we have seen throughout this book, nutritional harmony promotes disease and cancer prevention. However, peace and harmony of the mind are also necessary for chronic disease and cancer prevention. Emotional stress, anxiety, depression and anger have been shown to increase the risk of developing Type 2 diabetes and heart disease (including heart attacks).[1,2,3,4] One study found that younger adults with depression had a 23% increased risk of developing diabetes.[2] Anger in and of itself poses a significant risk to health. For example, in a large study with 13,000 participants, the participants with the highest levels of anger (but normal blood pressures) were twice as likely to develop heart disease and nearly three times as likely to have a heart attack or die from heart disease.[5] Anger has also been associated with an increased of risk prostate, colon and lung cancers.[6] A meta-analysis of 165 studies, found that people who were more prone to stress or who had difficulty coping with stress were more likely to develop cancer and also more likely to die from cancer.[7] Stress and mood disorders also impact survival with one study demonstrating that cancer patients who reported symptoms of depression died earlier than those cancer patients who had no symptoms of depression.[8] Thus, it is critical to address mental health and reestablish harmony of the mind in order to prevent the negative consequences associated with stress and mood disorders.

Nutritional deficiencies such as iron deficiency and vitamin D deficiency can contribute to mood disorders. The "magic trio" of B vitamins, magnesium, and omega-3 fatty acids significantly impact mood. Omega-3 fatty acids have been shown to help improve symptoms in ADHD, bipolar disorder, and anxiety.[9,10,11,12] Many studies have demonstrated that people who consume more omega-3 fatty acids as well as people with higher blood levels of omega-3 fatty acids have less depression than those who consume less omega-3 fatty acids.[13,14]

In order to understand the connection between mood disorders and nutrition, it is helpful to have a basic understanding of how the neurotransmitters responsible for mood are formed. Neurotransmitters are the chemicals in the brain that transmit information between neurons (nerve cells). The harmony and balance of these neurotransmitters is essential for maintaining mental health. For example, low levels of GABA and high levels of norepinephrine are associated with anxiety while low levels of serotonin are associated with depression. Many of the medications used to treat mood disorders are serotonin reuptake inhibitors. These medications increase the concentration of serotonin by preventing the serotonin from being taken back up into the neurons. Serotonin is formed from the precursors tryptophan and 5-HTP. **Some of the nutritional factors that impact the formation of serotonin include magnesium, B vitamins, calcium, iron, and zinc. Vitamin B6 and zinc are also necessary for the formation of GABA.** As we discussed earlier, our current diet depletes many of these vitamins and nutrients.

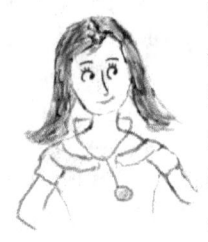 Foods that are high in the precursor tryptophan can improve mood by increasing the amount of serotonin formed. **Some of the foods highest in tryptophan include sacha inchi seeds, sesame seeds, sunflower seeds, pumpkin seeds, beans, oats, and spinach.**

Serotonin Formation

Tryptophan	->->->	5HTP	->->->	Serotonin
	Folate (B9)	Zinc		
	Iron	Magnesium		
	Calcium	Vitamin C		
	Vitamin B3	Vitamin B6		

In addition to foods, many teas also have been shown to be effective for anxiety and contain anticancer phytochemicals. As we have seen, the catechins in green tea have tremendous health and anticancer properties. Green tea also contains l-theanine which is an amino acid that increases GABA levels in the brain and promotes relaxation and improves mood. In a large study in Japan, the use of green tea was found to improve anxiety by 20%.[15] Chamomile tea has a sedative-like effect, often helping to relieve insomnia. Both chamomile and passionflower teas contain the anticancer phytochemical apigenin which, in vitro, has demonstrated anticancer activity against numerous cancers including breast, prostate, colon, ovarian, cervical and lung cancer cells.[16]

In addition to relieving anxiety and fighting cancer, the harmony of the phytochemicals in tea also provides other health benefits. For example, Lemon balm is not only calming, but has also been shown to improve memory, concentration and attention. [17] Holy basil is an adaptogenic herb. (Adaptogenic herbs have many health benefits and help the body deal with stress.) In addition to having a calming effect, Holy basil also helps regulate blood sugar in people with Type 2 diabetes.[18]

Conclusion

The most effective way to achieve optimum health is by finding balance and establishing harmony. Nutritional harmony and harmony of the mind are both critical components. They are interdependent such that an imbalance or discord in one naturally affects the other. As we have seen, the health of the gastrointestinal tract has a direct impact on the development of chronic disease and cancer. Leaky gut and bacterial imbalance not only affect nutrient absorption but also lead to chronic inflammation. Processed foods, sugar, excess omega-6 fatty acids, and artificial trans fats further contribute to this inflammation. This chronic inflammation as well as deficiencies in vitamin D and the "magic trio" (magnesium, omega-3 fatty acids, and B vitamins) contribute to diabetes, heart disease, cancer, neurodegenerative disease, and mood disorders. The consumption of whole foods can help prevent many chronic diseases and cancer. The harmony among the phytochemicals, minerals and vitamins in whole foods is responsible for their antioxidant, anti-inflammatory and anticancer activity. These health benefits cannot be duplicated by consuming any one component alone. Nutritional harmony also occurs when whole foods are combined often leading to synergy in which the combination has a greater impact on health than the sum of their individual effects. It is this remarkable power of whole foods, this nutritional harmony, and harmony of the mind which is our greatest defense against chronic disease and cancer.

Author's Note

My journey towards disease prevention and wellness began not long after I began practicing medicine. I found myself growing increasingly concerned by the number of young patients developing chronic diseases such as heart disease, diabetes, mood disorders and cancer. As I began to study Integrative Medicine, it became clear that the answer lies largely in food. I now focus on teaching patients how to prevent disease by providing them with information about nutrition and lifestyle changes. The focus of this book is nutrition but true health and well being can only be achieved by addressing all aspects of health including mind, body, and spirit. As a physician, there is no greater reward than seeing the health of your patients improve. Practicing medicine is truly a privilege for which I am grateful. I would like to thank you for taking the time to read *Nutritional Harmony* and hope that it helps you understand how food truly is medicine.

Sincerely,
Christine Fall, MD, ABIHM
Founder and President, L&D Integrative Medicine Consulting, LLC

Glossary

angiogenesis: the creation of new blood vessels

antioxidant: substances that protect the body from being damaged by free radicals by blocking the effects of free radicals

free radicals: reactive molecules that have an unpaired electron that can damage DNA or other parts of a cell; some sources include cigarette smoke, pollutants, pesticides, and inflammation

heme iron: iron that comes from an animal

in vitro study: study conducted outside of a living organism such as a study on cells in a test tube

in vivo study: study conducted on a living thing (such as humans, other animals or plants)

meta-analysis study: a study that analyzes results from many different studies and combines them using statistical analysis to come to a conclusion

metastasis: the spread of cancer to a site other than where it originated from neurodegenerative disease: disease that leads to progressive damage to the brain

non-heme iron: iron that comes from a plant

phytochemicals: substances from plants which provide health benefits

Sources

Chapter 1: Understanding Nutritional Harmony

[1] The Concise Oxford Dictionary of English Etymology in English Language Reference accessed via Oxford Reference Online (24 February 2007)

Chapter 2: A Healty Gastrointestinal Tract

[1] Possemiers S, Marzorati M, Verstraete W, Van de Wiele T., Bacteria and chocolate: a successful combination for probiotic delivery. J Food Microbiol. 2010 Jun 30;141(1-2):97-103.

Chapter 3: Nutrients that Impact Chronic Disease

[1] Wilson SM, Bivins BN, Russell KA, Bailey LB. Oral contraceptive use: impact on folate, vitamin B_6, and vitamin B_{12} status. Nutr Rev. 2011 Oct;69(10):572-83.

[2] A Daley CA, Abbott A et al., A review of fatty acid profiles and antioxidant content in grass-fed and grain-fed beef. Nutr J. 2010; 9:10.

[3] Pariza MW, Park Y & Cook ME. Conugated linoleic acid and the control of cancer and obesity. Toxicol. Sci. (1999) 52 (suppl 1): 107-110.

[4] Chen GC, Pang Z, Liu QF. Magnesium intake and risk of colorectal cancer: a meta-analysis of prospective stud-

ies. Eur J Clin Nutr. 2012 Nov;66(11):1182-6.

[5] Schöttker B, Jorde R2, Peasey A3, Thorand B et al., vitamin D and mortality: meta-analysis of individual participant data from a large consortium of cohort studies from Europe and the United States. BMJ 2014;348:g3656.

[6] Anglin RE, Samaan Z, Walter SD, McDonald SD. Vitamin D deficiency and depression in adults: systematic review and meta-analysis. Br J Psychiatry. 2013;202:100-107.

[7] Forman JP, Curhan GC, Taylor EN. Plasma 25-hydroxyvitamin D levels and risk of incident hypertension. Hypertension. 2007 May;49(5):1063-9.

[8] Littlejohns TJ , Henley WE, Lang IA, Annweiler C, et al., vitamin D and the risk of dementia and Alzheimer disease. Neurology, 2014 Sep 2;83(10):920-8.

[9] Churilla TM, Lesko SL, Brereton HD, et al. Serum vitamin D levels among patients in a clinical oncology practice compared to primary care patients in the same community: a case–control study. BMJ Open 2011;1:e000397

[10] Giovannucci E, Liu Y, Rimm EB, et al. Prospective study of predictors of vitamin D status and cancer incidence and mortality in men. J Natl Cancer Inst. 2006;98(7):451-459.

[11] Garland CF, Garland FC, Gorham ED, et al. The role of vitamin D in cancer prevention. Am J Public Health. 2006;96(2):252-261.

[12] Geleijnse JM, Vermeer C, Grobbee DE, Schurgers LJ, et al., Dietary intake of menaquinone is associated with a reduced risk of coronary heart disease: the Rotterdam Study. J Nutr. 2004 Nov;134(11):3100-5.

[13] Nimptsch K, Rohrmann S, Kaaks R, Linseisen J, Dietary vitamin K intake in relation to cancer incidence and mortality: results from the Heidelberg cohort of the European Prospective Investigation into Cancer and Nutrition (EPIC-Heidelberg). AmJ Clin Nutr. 2010 May;91(5):1348-58.

[14] Elder SJ, Haytowitz DB, Howe J, Peterson JW, Booth SL. Vitamin K contents of meat, dairy and fast food in the U.S. diet. Journal of Agricultural and Food Chemistry. 2006 Jan; 54(2): 463-467.

Chapter 4: Cancer

[1] Puangsombat K, Smith JS. Inhibition of heterocyclic amine formation in beef patties by ethanolic extracts of rosemary. J Food Sci. 2010;75(2):T40-47.

[2] Gibis M., Effect of oil marinades with garlic, onion, and lemon juice on the formation of heterocyclic aromatic amines in fried beef patties.J Agric Food Chem. 2007 Dec 12;55(25):10240-7.

[3] Omaye ST., Food and Nutritional Toxicology. CRC Press, 2004, Print.

[4] Knize MG, Felton JS. Formation and human risk of carcinogenic heterocyclic amines formed from natural precursors in meat. Nutr Rev. 2005 May;63(5):158-65.

[5] Puangsombat K, Gadgil P, Houser TA, Hunt MC, Smith JS. Occurrence of heterocyclic amines in cooked meat products. Meat Sci. 2012 Mar;90(3):739-46.

[6] The Five Worst Foods To Grill. Physicians Committee For Responsible Medicine website. July 3, 2010; http://www.pcrm.org/health/reports/the-five-worst-foods-to-grill

[7] Guo D & Dashwood R, Inhibition of 2-amino-3-me-

thylimidazo [4,5-f]quinoline (IQ)- DNA binding in rats given chlorophyllin: dose–response and time –course studies in the liver and colon. Carcinogenesis,1994; 15(4):763-66.

[8] Murray S, Lake BG, Gray S et al., Effect of cruciferous vegetable consumption on heterocyclic aromatic amine metabolism in man. Carcinogenesis (2001) 22 (9):1413-1420.

[9] Jakszyn P, Gonzalez CA. Nitrosamine and related food intake and gastric and oesophageal cancer risk: a systematic review of the epidemiological evidence. World J Gastroenterol. 2006 Jul 21;12(27):4296-303.

[10] Farhadian A, Jinap SN, Faridah A et al., Effects of marinating on the formation of polycyclic aromatic hydrocarbons (benzo[a]pyrene, benzo[b]fluoranthene and fluoranthene) in grilled beef meat. Food Control Volume 28, Issue 2, December 2012, pgs.420–425.

[11] Haorah J, Zhou L, Wang X, Xu G, Mirvish SS. Determination of total N-nitroso compounds and their precursors in frankfurters, fresh meat, dried salted fish, sauces, tobacco, and tobacco smoke particulates. J Agric Food Chem. 2001 Dec;49(12):6068-78.

[12] Akopyan G, Bonavida B. Understanding tobacco smoke carcinogen NNK and lung tumorigenesis. Int J Oncol. 2006 Oct;29(4):745-52.

[13] L. Santarelli RL, Pierre F, &Corpet DE.Processed meat and colorectal cancer: a review of epidemiologic and experimental evidence. Nutr Cancer. 2008; 60 (2):131-144.

[14] Nöthlings U, Lynne R. Wilkens LR, et al., Meat and Fat Intake as Risk Factors for Pancreatic Cancer: The Multiethnic Cohort Study.NCI J Natl Cancer Inst 2005 Oct; 97 (19): 1458-1465.

[15] Li F, An S, Hou L, Chen P, Lei C, Tan W. Red and processed meat intake and risk of bladder cancer: a meta-analysis.Int J Clin Exp Med. 2014 Aug 15;7(8):2100-10.

[16] Tsugane S, Sasazuki S. Diet and the risk of gastric cancer: review of epidemiological evidence. Gastric Cancer. 2007;10(2):75-83.

[17] Park Y, Spiegelman D, Hunter DJ, et al. Intakes of vitamins A, C, and E and use of multiple vitamin supplements and risk of colon cancer: a pooled analysis of prospective cohort studies. Cancer Causes Control. 2010;21(11):1745-1757.

[18] Pollak MN, Schernhammer ES & Hankinson SE. Insulin-like growth factors and neoplasia. Nature Reviews Cancer 2004 July; 4: 505-518

[19] Huang Y, Cai X et al., Prediabetes and the risk of cancer: a meta-analysis. Diabetologia 2014 Nov;57(11):2261-9.

[20] Suez J. Korem T, Zeevi D, et al., Artificial sweeteners induce glucose intolerance by altering the gut microbiota.Nature 2014 Oct 9;514(7521):181-6.

[21] Noda K, Nakayama K, Oku T. Serum glucose and insulin levels and erythritol balance after oral administration of erythritol in healthy subjects. Eur J Clin Nutr. 1994 Apr;48(4):286-9.

[22] Flint N, Naomi H, et al., Effects of Erythritol on Endothelial Function in Patients with Type 2 Diabetes Mellitus – A Pilot Study. Acta Diabetol. Jun 2014; 51(3): 513–516.

[23] Yasukawa K, Kitanaka S, Seo S. Inhibitory effect of stevioside on tumor promotion by 12-O-tetradecanoylphorbol-13-acetate in two-stage carcinogenesis in mouse skin. Biol Pharm Bull. 2002 Nov;25(11):1488-90.

[24] Boonkaewwan C, Toskulkao C, Vongsakul M. Anti-inflammatory and immunomodulatory activities of stevioside and steviol on colonic epithelial cells.J Sci Food Agric. 2013 Dec;93(15):3820-5.

[25] Scheid MM, Genaro PS, Moreno YM, Pastore GM. Freeze-dried powdered yacon: effects of FOS on serum glucose, lipids and intestinal transit in the elderly. Eur J Nutr. 2014 Oct;53(7):1457-64.

[26] Genta S, Cabrera W, Habib N, Pons J, Carillo IM, Grau A, Sánchez S. Yacon syrup: beneficial effects on obesity and insulin resistance in humans .Clin Nutr. 2009 Apr;28(2):182-7.

[27] Lin J , Zhang M, Song F, et al., Association between C-reactive protein and pre-diabetic status in a Chinese Han clinical population. Diabetes Metab Res Rev. 2009 Mar;25(3):219-23.

[28] Ridker PM, Buring JE, et al., Comparison of C-Reactive Protein and Low-Density Lipoprotein Cholesterol Levels in the Prediction of First Cardiovascular Events .N Engl J Med 2002 Nov; 347:1557-1565

Chapter 5: Food as Medicine

Cancer Prevention

[1] Block G, Patterson B, Subar A: Fruit, vegetables, and cancer prevention: a review of the epidemiological evidence. Nutr Cancer 1992, 18:1-29

[2] Ornish D, Weidner G, Fair WR, et al.Intensive lifestyle changes may affect the progression of prostate cancer. J Urol. 2005 Sep;174(3):1065-9

[3] June M Chan JM, Stampfer MD, Jing Ma, et al., Dairy products, calcium, and prostate cancer risk in the Phy-

sicians' Health Study. Am J Clin Nutr 2001 Oct;74 (4):549-554

[4] Giovannucci E, Ascherio A, Rimm EB, et al., Intake of carotenoids and retinol in relation to risk of prostate cancer.J Natl Cancer Inst. 1995 Dec 6;87(23):1767-76.

[5] Pantuck AJ, Leppert JT, Zomorodian N, et al., Phase II study of pomegranate juice for men with rising prostate-specific antigen following surgery or radiation for prostate cancer. Clin Cancer Res. 2006 Jul 1;12(13):4018-26.

[6] Demark-Wahnefried W, Polascik TJ, George SL et al., Flaxseed supplementation (not dietary fat restriction) reduces prostate cancer proliferation rates in men presurgery. Cancer Epidemiol Biomarkers Prev. 2008 Dec;17(12):3577-87

[7] Farvid MS, Cho E, Chen WY, Eliassen AH, Willett WC.Dietary protein sources in early adulthood and breast cancer incidence: prospective cohort study. BMJ. 2014 Jun 10;348:g3437

[8] Gunter MJ ,Hoover DR, et al., Insulin, Insulin-Like Growth Factor-I, and Risk of Breast Cancer in Postmenopausal Women. J Natl Cancer Inst. Jan 7, 2009; 101(1): 48–60

[9] Liu X, Lv K .Cruciferous vegetables intake is inversely associated with risk of breast cancer: a meta-analysis. Breast. 2013 Jun;22(3):309-13.

[10] Dongyan Y, Richard N. Baumgartner RN, et al., Dietary Intake of Folate, B-vitamins and Methionine and Breast Cancer Risk among Hispanic and Non-Hispanic White Women.PLoS One. 2013; 8(2): e54495

[11] Yang CY, Chiu HF, Cheng MF, Hsu TY, Cheng MF, Wu TN. Calcium and magnesium in drinking water and

the risk of death from breast cancer. J Toxicol Environ Health A. 2000 Jun;60(4):231-41.

[12] Kim J, Lim SY, Shin A, Sung MK, Ro J, Kang HS, Lee KS, Kim SW, Lee ES. Fatty fish and fish omega-3 fatty acid intakes decrease the breast cancer risk: a case-control study. BMC Cancer. 2009 Jun 30;9:216.

[13] Ghadirian P, Narod S, Fafard E, Costa M, Robidoux A, Nkondjock A. Breast cancer risk in relation to the joint effect of BRCA mutations and diet diversity. Breast Cancer Res Treat. 2009 Sep;117(2):417-22.

[14] Pierce JP, Stefanick ML, et al., Greater Survival After Breast Cancer in Physically Active Women With High Vegetable-Fruit Intake Regardless of Obesity.

Alliums

[1] Boivin D, Lamy S, Lord-Dufour, et al., Antiproliferative and antioxidant activities of common vegetables: A comparative study. Food Chem., 112(2):374{380, 2009.

[2] Yang J, Meyers KJ, Van der Heide J, Liu RH. Varietal differences in phenolic content and antioxidant and antiproliferative activities of onions. J Agric Food Chem. 2004 Nov 3;52(22):6787-93.

[3] Larson A et al., Therapeutic potential of quercetin to decrease blood pressure: review of efficacy and mechanisms. Advances in Nutrition 2012 Jan; 3(1):39-46.

[4] Patil BS, Leonard M. Pike LM , & Yo KS. Variation in the Quercetin Content in Different Colored Onions (Allium cepa L.) J. Amer Soc. Hort. Sci. 120(6):909-913. 1995.

[5] Cheng A, Chen X, Jin Q, et al., Comparison of Phenolic Content and Antioxidant Capacity of Red and Yel-

low Onions. Czech J. Food Sci. Vol. 31, 2013, No. 5: 501–508.

[6] Jiménez-Monreal AM, García-Diz L, Martínez-Tomé M, Mariscal M, Murcia MA. Influence of cooking methods on antioxidant activity of vegetables. J Food Sci. 2009 Apr;74(3):H97-H103.

[7] USDA Database for the Flavonoid Content of Selected Foods, Release 2.1 (2007); www.ImmuneHealthScience.com

[8] Zakarova A, Seo JY, Kim HY, et al., Garlic sprouting is associated with increased antioxidant activity and concomitant changes in the metabolite profile.J Agric Food Chem. 2014 Feb 26;62(8):1875-80

Cruciferous Vegetables

[1] Zhang CX, Ho SC, Chen YM, Fu JH, Cheng SZ, Lin FY. Greater vegetable and fruit intake is associated with a lower risk of breast cancer among Chinese women.Int J Cancer. 2009 Jul 1;125(1):181-8

[2] Cohen JH, Kristal AR, Stanford JL, Fruit and vegetable intakes and prostate cancer risk. J Natl Cancer Inst. 2000 Jan 5;92(1):61-8.

[3] Zhang X, Shu XO, Xiang YB, Yang G, Li H, Gao J, Cai H, Gao YT, Zheng W. Cruciferous vegetable consumption is associated with a reduced risk of total and cardiovascular disease mortality. Am J Clin Nutr. 2011 Jul; 94(1):240-246

[4] McNaughton SA, Marks GC. Development of a food composition database for the estimation of dietary intakes of glucosinolates, the biologically active constituents of cruciferous vegetables. Journal of Nutrition 2003, 90(3): 687–697

Carrots

[1] Kobaek-Larsen M, Christensen LP, Vach W, Ritskes-Hoitinga J, Brandt K. Inhibitory effects of feeding with carrots or (-)-falcarinol on development of azoxymethane-induced preneoplastic lesions in the rat colon. J Agric Food Chem. 2005 Mar 9;53(5):1823-7.

[2] Oude Griep LM, Verschuren WM, Kromhout D, Ocké MC, Geleijnse JM. Colours of fruit and vegetables and 10-year incidence of CHD. British Journal of Nutrition 2011 Nov; 11 106 (10): 1562-1569.

[3] Metzger BT & Barnes DM. Diversity of anti-inflammatory polyacetylenes in colored carrots (Daucus carota L.) FASEB J 2009 April; 899.1

[4] Imsic M, Winkler S, Tomkins B, Jones R. Effect of storage and cooking on beta-carotene isomers in carrots (Daucus carota L. cv. 'Stefano'). J Agric Food Chem. 2010 Apr 28;58(8):5109-13.

Spinach

[1] Castenmiller JJ, West CE, Linssen JP, van het Hof KH, Voragen AG. The food matrix of spinach is a limiting factor in determining the bioavailability of beta-carotene and to a lesser extent of lutein in humans.J Nutr. 1999 Feb;129(2):349-55.

[2] Castenmiller JJ, van de Poll CJ, West CE, Brouwer IA, Thomas CM, van Dusseldorp M. Bioavailability of folate from processed spinach in humans. Effect of food matrix and interaction with carotenoids. Ann Nutr Metab. 2000;44(4):163-9.

[3] Ribaya-Mercado JD, Blumberg JB.Lutein and zeaxanthin and their potential roles in disease prevention.J Am Coll Nutr. 2004 Dec;23(6 Suppl):567S-587S.

[4] Lester GE, Makus DJ, Hodges DM, Relationship between fresh-packaged spinach leaves exposed to continuous light or dark and bioactive contents: effects of cultivar, leaf size, and storage duration. J Agric Food Chem. 2010 Mar 10;58(5):2980-7

Fruits

[1] Sun J, Chu YF, Wu X, Liu RH. Antioxidant and antiproliferative activities of common fruits. J. Agric. Food. Chem. 2002 50(25):7449–7454.

[2] Hakim IA, Harris RB, Ritenbaugh Citrus peel use is associated with reduced risk of squamous cell carcinoma of the skin. Nutr Cancer. 2000;37(2):161-8.

Apples

[1] Reagan-Shaw S, Eggert D, Mukhtar H, Ahmad N. Antiproliferative effects of apple peel extract against cancer cells. Nutr Cancer. 2010;62(4):517-24.

[2] Chai SC, Hooshmand S, Raz L Saadat RL , Arjmandi BH. Daily apple consumption promotes cardiovascular health in postmenopausal women. The FASEB Journal. 2011;25:971.10

[3] Huber GM, Rupasinghe HP. Phenolic profiles and antioxidant properties of apple skin extracts. J. Food Sci. 74(9):693, 2009.

[4] Boyer J, Liu RH. Apple phytochemicals and their health benefits.Nutr J. 2004; 3: 5.

Citrus Fruits

[1] Song JK, Bae JM. Citrus fruit intake and breast cancer risk: a quantitative systematic review. J Breast Cancer.

2013 Mar;16(1):72-6.

2) Benavente-García O, Castillo J.Update on uses and properties of citrus flavonoids: new findings in anticancer, cardiovascular, and anti-inflammatory activity. J Agric Food Chem. 2008 Aug 13;56(15):6185-205.

3) Cassidy A, Rimm EB, O'Reilly EJ, Logroscino G, Kay C, Chiuve SE, Rexrode KM.Dietary flavonoids and risk of stroke in women.Stroke. 2012 Apr;43(4):946-51.

4) Lee CJ, Wilson L, Jordan MA, Nguyen V, Tang J, Smiyun G. Hesperidin suppressed proliferations of both human breast cancer and androgen-dependent prostate cancer cells.Phytother Res. 2010 Jan;24 Suppl 1:S15-9.

5) Omidbaigi R, Nasiri MF, Sadr ZB. Hesperidin in citrus species, quantitative distribution during fruit maturation and optimal harvesting time. Acta Hort. 2002(ISHS) 576:91-97

6) Peterson JJ, Gary R, Beecherb GR, Bhagwatc SA, et al., Flavanones in grapefruit, lemons, and limes: A compilation and review of the data from the analytical literature. Journal of Food Composition and Analysis 19 (2006) S74–S80.

7) Bharti S, Rani N, Krishnamurthy B, Arya DS. Preclinical evidence for the pharmacological actions of naringin: a review. Planta Med. 2014 Apr;80(6):437-51.

8) Hasegawa S, Lam LKT, Miller EG. Citrus limonoids biochemistry and possible importance in Human Nutrition. Fereidoon Shahidi, Chi-Tang Ho ed. Phytochemicals and Phytopharmaceuticals: The American Oil Chemists Society, 2000

Berries

[1] Wu X, Beecher GR , Holden JM, et al.,Concentrations of Anthocyanins in Common Foods in the United States and Estimation of Normal Consumption.J. Agric. Food Chem., 2006, 54 (11), pp 4069–4075

[2] Wang LS, Sardo C, Rocha CM, McIntyre CM, Frankel W, Arnold M, Martin E, Lechner JF, Stoner GD. Effect of freeze-dried black raspberries on human colorectal cancer lesions. AACR Special Conference in Cancer Research. Advances in Colon Cancer Research; 2007. #B31.

[3] Elaine M. Daniel EM, Alexander S. Krupnick AS, Young-Hun Heur YH, et al. Extraction, stability, and quantitation of ellagic acid in various fruits and nuts. Journal of Food Composition and Analysis 1989 Dec; 2 (4): 338-349.

[4] Udani JK, Singh BB, et al.,Effects of Açai (Euterpe oleracea Mart.) berry preparation on metabolic parameters in a healthy overweight population: A pilot study Nutr J. 2011; 10: 45.

[5] Hoggard N, Cruickshank M, Moar KM, et al., A single supplement of a standardised bilberry (Vaccinium myrtillus L.) extract (36 % wet weight anthocyanins) modifies glycaemic response in individuals with type 2 diabetes controlled by diet and lifestyle.J Nutr Sci. 2013 Jul 24;2:e22

[6] Akhtar MS, Ramzan A, Ali A, Ahmad M.Effect of Amla fruit (Emblica officinalis Gaertn.) on blood glucose and lipid profile of normal subjects and type 2 diabetic patients. Int J Food Sci Nutr. 2011 Sep;62(6):609-16.

[7] Oszmian J, Wojdy A, Kolniak J. Effect of L-ascorbic acid, sugar, pectin and freeze–thaw treatment on polyphenol content of frozen strawberries. LWT–Food Sci-

ence and Technology 42 (2009) 581–586

[8] Michalczyk M, Macura R & Matsuszak. The effect of air drying, freeze -drying, and storage on the quality and antioxidant activity of some selected berries. Journal of Food Processing and Preservation 2009 Feb; 33 (1): 11-21.

[9] Tiffany J. Hager. Processing Effects on the Antioxidant Capacity, Polyphenolic Content, Absorption and Metabolism of Apache Blackberries. Chapter 6 Effects of processing and storage on the ellagitannin composition. ProQuest, 2007

[10] Grace MH, Massey AR, Mbeunkui F, Yousef GG, Lila MA. Comparison of health-relevant flavonoids in commonly consumed cranberry products. J Food Sci. 2012 Aug;77(8):H176-83

Tomatoes

[1] U.S. Department of Agriculture, Agricultural Research Service. 2010. USDA National Nutrient Database for Standard Reference, Release 24. Nutrient Data Laboratory Home Page, www.ars.usda.gov/ba/bhnrc/ndl

[2] Perkins-Veazie P, Collins JK, D Pair SD, and Robert W. Lycopene content differs among red-fleshed watermelon cultivars. Journal of the Science of Food and Agriculture 2001 Aug; 81 (10): 983-987

[3] Tomatoes and Tomato Products: Nutritional, Medicinal and Therapeutic Properties.Chapter 6 Antioxidant Activity in Tomato: A Function of Genotype Authors Kaur C and Kapoor HC. CRC Press, Jan 9, 2008

[4] Sharma, S.K. and Maguer M.L. Lycopene in tomatoes and tomato pulp. Ital. J. Food Sci. 1996; 2: 107-113.

[5] Dewanto V, Wu X, Adom KK, Liu RH. Thermal processing enhances the nutritional value of tomatoes by increasing total antioxidant activity.J Agric Food Chem. 2002 May 8;50(10):3010-4.

Avocados

[1] Slater G et al. Seasonal variation in the composition of California avocados. J. Agric. Food Chem., 1975, 23 (3), pp 468–474

Legumes

[1] Adebamowo C. A. et al. Dietary flavonols and flavonol-rich foods intake and the risk of breast cancer. Int J Cancer 2005;114(4):628-633.

[2] Zanovec M. et al., Comparison of Nutrient Density and Nutrient-to-Cost between Cooked and Canned Beans. Food Nutr Sci. 2011 2(2):66-73.

Nuts

[1] U.S. Department of Agriculture, Agricultural Research Service. 2010. USDA National Nutrient Database for Standard Reference, Release 23. Nutrient Data Laboratory Home Page, http://www.ars.usda.gov/ba/bhnrc/ndl

[2] U.S. Department of Agriculture, Agricultural Research Service. 2010. USDA National Nutrient Database for Standard Reference, Release 27. Nutrient Data Laboratory Home Page, http://www.ars.usda.gov/ba/bhnrc/ndl

[3] Hu FB, Stampfer MJ, et al., Frequent nut consumption and risk of coronary heart disease in women: prospective cohort study. BMJ. Nov 14, 1998; 317(7169): 1341–1345.

[4] Albert CM, Gaziano JM, Willett WC, Manson JE. Nut consumption and decreased risk of sudden cardiac death in the Physicians' Health Study.Arch Intern Med. 2002 Jun 24;162(12):1382-7.

[5] Bao Y, Han J, Hu FB, Giovannucci EL, Stampfer MJ, Willett WC, Fuchs CS. Association of nut consumption with total and cause-specific mortality.N Engl J Med. 2013 Nov 21;369(21):2001-11.

[6] Jiang R, Manson JE, Stampfer MJ, Liu S, Willett WC, Hu FB. Nut and peanut butter consumption and risk of type 2 diabetes in women. JAMA. 2002;288(20):2554-2560.

[7] Bes-Rastrollo M, Wedick NM. Prospective study of nut consumption, long-term weight change, and obesity risk in women.Am J Clin Nutr. Jun 2009; 89(6): 1913–1919

Walnuts

[1] Yang J, Liu RH, Halim L. Antioxidant and antiproliferative activities of common edible nut seeds. Food Science and Technology 2009 42:1-8.

[2] Fitschen PJ, Rolfhus KR, Winfrey MR, Allen BK, Manzy M, Maher MA. Cardiovascular effects of consumption of black versus English walnuts. J Med Food. 2011 Sep;14(9):890-8.

[3] Cosmulescu S, Trandafir I, et al., Phenolics of Green Husk in Mature Walnut Fruits.Not. Bot. Hort. Agrobot. Cluj 38 (1) 2010, 53-56.

[4] Hardman WE. Walnuts have potential for cancer prevention and treatment in mice.J Nutr. 2014 Apr;144(4 Suppl):555S-560S.

[5] Hardman WE, Ion G.. Suppression of implanted MDA-

MB 231 human breast cancer growth in nude mice by dietary walnut.Nutr Cancer. 2008;60(5):666-74.

[6] Russel J. Reiter, Dun-Xian Tan, Lucien C. Manchester, Ahmet Korkmaz, Lorena Fuentes-Broto, W. Elaine Hardman, Sergio A. Rosales-Corral, Wenbo Qi. A Walnut-Enriched Diet Reduces the Growth of LNCaP Human Prostate Cancer Xenografts in Nude Mice. Cancer Investigation, 2013; 31.

Almonds

[1] Platt ID, Josse AR, Kendall CW, Jenkins DJ, El-Sohemy A. Postprandial effects of almond consumption on human osteoclast precursors—an ex vivo study. Metabolism. 2011 Jul;60(7):923-9.

Pistachios

[1] U.S. Department of Agriculture, Agricultural Research Service. 2010. USDA National Nutrient Database for Standard Reference, Release 27. Nutrient Data Laboratory Home Page, http://www.ars.usda.gov/ba/bhnrc/ndl

[2] Phillips KM, Ruggio DM, Ashraf-Khorassani M. Phytosterol composition of nuts and seeds commonly consumed in the United States.J Agric Food Chem. 2005 Nov 30;53(24):9436-45.

[3] Aldemir M, Okulu E, Neselioglu S, Erel O, Kayıgil O.Pistachio diet improves erectile function parameters and serum lipid profiles in patients with erectile dysfunction.Int J Impot Res. 2011 Jan-Feb;23(1):32-8.

Brazil nuts

[1] Dennert G et al.,Selenium for preventing cancer. Cochrane Database Syst Rev 2011:CD005195.

Top Ranking Nuts

[1] U.S.Department of Agriculture, Agricultural Research Service. 2010. USDA National Nutrient Database for Standard Reference, Release 27. Nutrient Data Laboratory Home Page, http://www.ars.usda.gov/ba/bhnrc/ndl

Seeds

Flaxseeds

[1] Chen J, Stavro PM, Thompson LU. Dietary flaxseed inhibits human breast cancer growth and metastasis and downregulates expression of insulin-like growth factor and epidermal growth factor receptor. Nutrition & Cancer. 2002;43:187-92.

[2] Lin X, Gingrich JR, Bao W, Li J, Haroon ZA, Demark-Wahnefried W. Effect of flaxseed supplementation on prostatic carcinoma in transgenic mice. Urology 2002;60:919-24.

[3] Dwivedi C, Natarajan K, Matthees DP. Chemopreventive effects of dietary flaxseed oil on colon tumor development. Nutr Cancer. 2005;51(1):52-8.

Chia Seeds

[1] Nieman D.C., et al. Chia Seed Supplementation and Disease Risk Factors in Overweight Women: A Metabolomics Investigation. The Journal of Alternative and Complementary Medicine. 2012;18(7):700-708

Mushrooms

[1] Schulzová V, Hajslová J, Peroutka R, Gry J, Andersson HC. Influence of storage and household processing on the agaritine content of the cultivated Agaricus mushroom. Food Addit Contam. 2002 Sep;19(9):853-62.

[2] Zhang M, Huang J, Xie X, Holman CD. Dietary intakes of mushrooms and green tea combine to reduce the risk of breast cancer in Chinese women. Int J Cancer. 2009 Mar 15;124(6):1404-8

[3] Ina K, Kataoka T, Ando T. The use of lentinan for treating gastric cancer. Anticancer Agents Med Chem. 2013 Jun;13(5):681-8.

Green tea

[1] Kuriyama S et al., Green tea consumption and mortality due to cardiovascular disease, cancer, and all causes in Japan: the Ohsaki study.JAMA. 2006 Sep 13;296(10):1255-65.

[2] Larsson S, Wolk A. Tea consumption and ovarian cancer risk in a population-based cohort. Arch Intern Med 2005;165(22): 2683-2686

[3] Sun CL, Yuan JM, Koh WP, Yu M., Green tea, black tea and breast cancer risk: a meta-analysis of epidemiological studies.Carcinogenesis 2006 Jul;27(7):1310-5.

[4] Kurahashi N, Sasazuki S, Motoki Iwasaki M, et al., Green Tea Consumption and Prostate Cancer Risk in Japanese Men: A Prospective Study. Am. J. Epidemiol. (2008) 167 (1): 71-77.

[5] Yang G, Shu XO, Li H, Chow WH, Ji BT, Zhang X, Gao YT, Zheng W. Prospective cohort study of green tea consumption and colorectal cancer risk in women.Cancer Epidemiol Biomarkers Prev. 2007 Jun;16(6):1219-23.

Herbs

Parsley

[1] Zheng GQ, Kenney PM, Lam LKT. Myristicin: a potential cancer chemopreventive agent from parsley leaf oil. J. Agric. Food Chem., 1992, 40 (1): 107–110

[2] Gates MA, Vitonis AF, et al., Flavonoid intake and ovarian cancer risk in a population-based case-control study. Int J Cancer. Apr 15, 2009; 124(8): 1918–1925.

Rosemary

[1] Yesil-Celiktas O, Sevimli C, Bedir E, Vardar-Sukan F. Inhibitory effects of rosemary extracts, carnosic acid and rosmarinic acid on the growth of various human cancer cell lines. Plant Foods Hum Nutr. 2010 Jun;65(2):158-63.

Turmeric Curcumin

[1] Yang F, Lim GP, Begum AN, Ubeda OJ, Simmons MR, Ambegaokar SS, et al. Curcumin inhibits formation of amyloid beta oligomers and fibrils, binds plaques, and reduces amyloid in vivo. J Biol Chem. 2005;280:5892–901

[2] Ono K, Hasegawa K, Naiki H, Yamada MJ. Curcumin has potent anti-amyloidogenic effects for Alzheimer's beta fibrils in vitro. Neurosci Res. 2004;75:742–50.

[3] Sanmukhani J, Satodia V, Trivedi J, et al., Efficacy and safety of curcumin in major depressive disorder: a randomized controlled trial.Phytother Res. 2014 Apr;28(4):579-85

[4] Kulkarni SK, Bhutani MK, Bishnoi M. Antidepres-

sant activity of curcumin: involvement of serotonin and dopamine system.)Psychopharmacology (Berl). 2008 Dec;201(3):435-42.

5) Boonla O, Kukongviriyapan U, Pakdeechote P, et al., Curcumin improves endothelial dysfunction and vascular remodeling in 2K-1C hypertensive rats by raising nitric oxide availability and reducing oxidative stress. Nitric Oxide. 2014 Sep 4;42C:44-53.

6) Ramirez-Tortosa MC, Mesa MD, Aguilera MC, Quiles JL, et al., Oral administration of a turmeric extract inhibits LDL oxidation and has hypocholesterolemic effects in rabbits with experimental atherosclerosis. Atherosclerosis. 1999;147:371–378.

7) Chandran B, Goel A. A randomized, pilot study to assess the efficacy and safety of curcumin in patients with active rheumatoid arthritis. Phytother Res. 2012 Nov;26(11):1719-25.

8) Nishiyama T, Mae T, Kishida H, Tsukagawa M et al., Curcuminoids and sesquiterpenoids in turmeric (Curcuma longa L.) suppress an increase in blood glucose level in type 2 diabetic KK-Ay mice. J Agric Food Chem. 2005;53:959–963

9) Anand P, Sundaram C, Jhurani S, Kunnumakkara AB, Aggarwal BB. Curcumin and cancer: An "old-age" disease with an "age-old" solution. Cancer Lett 2008 Aug 18;267(1):133-64

10) Kunnumakkara AB, Anand P, Aggarwal BB. Curcumin inhibits proliferation, invasion, angiogenesis and metastasis of different cancers through interaction with multiple cell signaling proteins. Cancer Lett 2008 Oct 8;269(2):199-225.

Food Synergy

[1] Canene-Adams K, Lindshield BL, Wang S, Jeffery EH, Clinton SK, Erdman JW Jr. Combinations of tomato and broccoli enhance antitumor activity in dunning r3327-h prostate adenocarcinomas. Cancer Res. 2007 Jan 15;67(2):836-43.

[2] Zhang M, Huang J, Xie X, Holman CD. Dietary intakes of mushrooms and green tea combine to reduce the risk of breast cancer in Chinese women. Int J Cancer. 2009 Mar 15;124(6):1404-8

[3] Chen W, Zhang Y, Tan N, Qi Y, Zhu JS,. Synergy of Ganoderma lucidum extract ReishiMax and green tea polyphenols Tegreen in anticancer in a S180-inoculation model. FASEB J. Meeting Abstracts, 2007, 21(6): Abstract# 852.3.

Chapter 6: Harmony of the Mind

[1] Pouwer F, Kupper N, Adriaanse MC. Does emotional stress cause type 2 diabetes mellitus? A review from the European Depression in Diabetes (EDID) Research Consortium. Discov Med. 2010 Feb;9(45):112-8.

[2] Brown LC, Majumdar SR, Newman SC, Johnson JA. History of depression increases risk of type 2 diabetes in younger adults.Diabetes Care. 2005 May;28(5):1063-7.

[3] Rozanski A, Blumenthal JA, Kaplan J. Impact of psychological factors on the pathogenesis of cardiovascular disease and implications for therapy. Circulation. 1999;99(16):2192-2217.

[4] Krantz DS, McCeney MK. Effects of psychological and social factors on organic disease: a critical assessment of research on coronary heart disease. Annu Rev Psychol. 2002;53:341-369.

[5] Williams JE, Paton CC, Siegler IC, Eigenbrodt ML, Nieto FJ, Tyroler HA. Anger proneness predicts coronary heart disease risk: prospective analysis from the atherosclerosis risk in communities (ARIC) study.Circulation. 2000 May 2;101(17):2034-9.

[6] White VM, English DR, Coates H, Lagerlund M, Borland R, Giles GG. Is cancer risk associated with anger control and negative affect? Findings from a prospective cohort study. Psychosom Med. 2007 Sep-Oct;69(7):667-74.

[7] Chida Y, Hamer M, Wardle J, Steptoe A. Do stress-related psychosocial factors contribute to cancer incidence and survival? Nat Clin Pract Oncol. 2008 Aug;5(8):466-75.

[8] Brown K.W. et al., Psychological distress and cancer survival: a follow-up 10 years after diagnosis. Psychosom Med. 2003 Jul-Aug;65(4):636-43

[9] Parker G, Gibson NA, Brotchie H, Heruc G, Rees AM, Hadzi-Pavlovic D. Omega-3 fatty acids and mood disorders. Am J Psychiatry. 2006 Jun;163(6):969-78.

[10] Bloch MH, Qawasmi A. Omega-3 fatty acid supplementation for the treatment of children with attention-deficit/hyperactivity disorder symptomatology: systematic review and meta-analysis. J Am Acad Child Adolesc Psychiatry. 2011 Oct;50(10):991-1000.

[11] Sarris J, Mischoulon D, Schweitzer I. Omega-3 for bipolar disorder: meta-analyses of use in mania and bipolar depression.J Clin Psychiatry. 2012 Jan;73(1):81-6.

[12] Kiecolt-Glaser JK, Belury MA, Andridge R, Malarkey WB, Glaser R. Omega-3 supplementation lowers inflammation and anxiety in medical students: a randomized controlled trial. Brain Behav Immun. 2011 Nov;25(8):1725-34

13) Colangelo LA, He K, Whooley MA, Daviglus ML, Liu K. Higher dietary intake of long-chain w-3 polyunsaturated fatty acids is inversely associated with depressive symptoms in women. Nutrition. 2009;25(10):1011–1019w

14) Panagiotakos DB, Mamplekou E, Pitsavos C, et al. Fatty acids intake and depressive symptomatology in a greek sample: an epidemiological analysis. Journal of the American College of Nutrition. 2010;29(6):586–594.

15) Hozawa A, Kuriyama S, Nakaya N, Green tea consumption is associated with lower psychological distress in a general population: the Ohsaki Cohort 2006 Study. Am J Clin Nutr (September 30, 2009).

16) Shukla S & Gupta S. Apigenin: A Promising Molecule for Cancer Prevention. Pharm Res. Jun 2010; 27(6): 962–978.

17) Kennedy DO, Wake G, Savelev S, Tildesley NT, Perry EK, Wesnes KA, Scholey AB.Modulation of mood and cognitive performance following acute administration of single doses of Melissa officinalis (Lemon balm) with human CNS nicotinic and muscarinic receptor-binding properties. Neuropsychopharmacology. 2003 Oct;28(10):1871-81.

18) Agrawal P, Rai V, Singh RB. Randomized placebo-controlled, single blind trial of holy basil leaves in patients with noninsulin-dependent diabetes mellitus.Int J Clin Pharmacol Ther. 1996 Sep;34(9):406-9.

www.ingramcontent.com/pod-product-compliance
Lightning Source LLC
Chambersburg PA
CBHW071215280526
45787CB00002B/693